how to Pass the CSA Exam

Imtiaz Ahmad
BSc (Hons) MBBS DRCOG FRCGP MSc Sports Med
MFSEM (UK) PGCertMedEd
GP Principal and Trainer at South Lambeth Road Practice, London
and Musculoskeletal Lead for Lambeth
Course Organiser for London MRCGP Courses

Raj Nair
BSc (Hons) MBBS FRCGP DCH DRCOG DFSRH PGCert
Training Programme Director
Guy's & St Thomas' GP Specialty Training Programme;
Associate Director of Postgradua┼ ┼┼┼┼┼
Guy's & St Thomas';
GP Principal and Trainer
Albion Street Group Practice
South East London

Martin Block
MA MBBS MRCGP
Programme Director, Imperial GP Specialty Training Programme
GP Principal and Trainer, Clapham Park Group Practice, London

Graham Easton
MBBS MSc FRCGP
Senior Clinical Teaching Fellow and Educational Supervisor,
Academic ST4 programme
Department of Primary Care and Public Health
Imperial College Medical School, London
GP Principal and Trainer, Ealing, London

T0356043

WILEY Blackwell

This edition first published 2015 © 2015 by John Wiley & Sons, Ltd.

Registered Office
John Wiley & Sons, Ltd., The Atrium, Southern Gate, Chichester, West Sussex, PO19 8SQ, UK

Editorial Offices
9600 Garsington Road, Oxford, OX4 2DQ, UK
The Atrium, Southern Gate, Chichester, West Sussex, PO19 8SQ, UK
350 Main Street, Malden, MA 02148-5020, USA

For details of our global editorial offices, for customer services and for information about how to apply for permission to reuse the copyright material in this book please see our website at www.wiley.com/wiley-blackwell

The right of the authors to be identified as the authors of this work has been asserted in accordance with the UK Copyright, Designs and Patents Act 1988.

Library of Congress Cataloging-in-Publication Data

Ahmad, Imtiaz (General practitioner) author.
    How to pass the CSA exam : for GP trainees and MRCGP CSA candidates / Imtiaz Ahmad, Raj Nair,
Martin Block, Graham Easton.
        p. ; cm.
    Includes index.
    ISBN 978-1-118-47101-2 (pbk.)
I. Nair, Raj (General practitioner), author.   II. Block, Martin (General practitioner), author.   III. Easton, Graham,
author.   IV. Title.
    [DNLM: 1. General Practice–methods–Great Britain.   2. Clinical Competence–standards–Great Britain.
3. Credentialing–Great Britain.   4. Test Taking Skills–Great Britain.   W 40 FA1]
    RC58
    616.0076–dc23
                                                    2014017312
A catalogue record for this book is available from the British Library.

Wiley also publishes its books in a variety of electronic formats. Some content that appears in print may
not be available in electronic books.

Cover images courtesy of the authors

Set in 8.5/12pt Helvetica by SPi Publisher Services, Pondicherry, India
Printed and bound in Singapore by Markono Print Media Pte Ltd

1   2015

Contents

Acknowledgements

We would like to thank several people who have been key to this book and DVD.

We are extremely grateful to our four 'trainees' who were happy to put themselves under the spotlight in the DVD consultations for the benefit of their colleagues who are preparing for the exam. They have also made really useful comments throughout the early chapters:

- **Dr Mydhili Chellappah**
- **Dr Sam Eden**
- **Dr Shaleen Ahmad**
- **Dr Murtaza Ali**

At the time of filming, Mydhili, Sam and Shaleen had all recently passed the CSA. Murtaza was preparing for it, so he made the most of the others' experience and the consultation practice with feedback. We are delighted to say that soon after filming the DVD, Murtaza passed the CSA – congratulations!

For the DVD we depended heavily on the professional expertise of our two actors who gave us a range of very convincing simulated patients in the consultations:

- **Melody Schroeder**
- **Hari Sajjan**

Thanks also to our production team who did a great job filming and editing the DVD:

- **Tom Durley:** tbcdurley@gmail.com
- **Jules Harding:** http://jgharding.com

We are also very grateful to the **South Lambeth Road Practice** for allowing us to use their premises for filming the DVD. A big thank you to colleagues, trainees, friends and families for help and support with this project.

Foreword

by Roger Neighbour OBE DSc MA FRCGP FRCP
Past President, Royal College of General Practitioners
Author of *The Inner Consultation*

At my time of life I feel entitled to the occasional rant. And when my good friend Graham Easton emailed me to ask if I would contribute a foreword to this book, I felt a rant coming on. Let me explain.

Aside from clinical practice, my career has had two strands, both of which I'm passionate about. The first is the process of the consultation, that choreographed conversation between patient and doctor which, skilfully and subtly performed, effectively matches doctor's resources to patient's needs, to the satisfaction of both. It has been my privilege to spend many years trying to help the rising generation of GPs discover the delight that comes from taking as much pride in the fluffy communication stuff of general practice as we do in mastering its biomedicine.

The second strand has been assessment, specifically the MRCGP exam. I – you – we all want to be proud of the medicine we practise, and it hurts us, individually and collectively, if the occasional less-than-competent colleague lets the side down. The setting and – yes – policing of the standards for entry to our discipline is part of how we guarantee our professional reputation. No one likes doing exams; but as an MRCGP examiner for twenty years and its chief examiner for five, I know how much thought has gone into developing an examination that tests all the things that matter in ways that everyone – College and candidates, public and politicians – can trust.

Unsurprisingly, with the passage of time both processes – the consultation and the assessment – have become industrialized. During your training you will have read books, studied models, made videos, done COTs, worked through online materials and gone on courses, all intended to help you – like the proverbial horse led to water – develop a thirst for consulting competence. But as always, with industrialization have come unintended consequences. The CSA, to my mind, strikes a sensible balance between the 'hard' physical and the 'soft' communication domains. Nevertheless, one recurring lament among MRCGP examiners is that some candidates are so preoccupied with pursuing a physical problem that they neglect to attend to the human being afflicted by it. Another complaint is that the consulting skills intended to support the doctor–patient interaction – laudable strategies such as 'exploring ideas, concerns and expectations', 'shared decision-making', 'checking for understanding' – are sometimes reduced to formulaic clichés, mouthed for their own sake rather than being the means to a genuinely patient-centred consultation. I remember once, in the days when the MRCGP exam had an oral component, being told by a candidate that he would 'ICE the patient, and all that rubbish'!

There is an exam preparation industry too. I've just Googled 'MRCGP exam preparation' and got 54,500 hits, of which 4,500 are about the CSA. That is hardly surprising. It's an expensive exam; the stakes are high and the chances of failure not negligible; and in this more than the other components of the MRCGP, your personal qualities are on the line. Small wonder, therefore, that you, the potential reader of this book, are an easy market for the purveyors of materials intended to boost your chances of success. But here again there are unintended consequences, this time the danger of perpetuating the myth that, to pass the CSA, something more than competence – some arcane secret, some privileged insight, some special formula – is required. Well, it isn't.

A Zen story is told of a pupil monk who went to see the master and asked, 'Master, how should I live perfectly?' The master replied, 'First make yourself perfect – and then live naturally.' By the same token, the way to pass the

CSA is to practise your consultations over the months of your training, gradually developing your clinical skills and your consulting style until they come naturally – and then, on the day of the exam, just do what you always do.

By now you can perhaps understand the rant that sprang to my lips when I received Graham Easton's email. This will be another book (I thought, before I read the manuscript) coaching the unprepared in how to play-act for the examiners and frightening them even more with the perfection of the case examples. 'I'm not sure this is a helpful approach,' I emailed back, 'as the written medium tends to lead candidates to think (wrongly) that good performance lies more in what they say and less in how they say it and how they relate to the patient. It often seems to have the effect of making the trainee talk more and listen less.'

How wrong I was. When I read the text, my spirits soared. These authors understand, I soon realized, that success in the CSA follows naturally from thoughtful, conscientious practice developed systematically through everyday contact with patients. They understand that consulting skills are the servant of the clinical process, not a distraction from it. They are on the same wavelength as that Zen master. To be sure, the information they give about how the exam works, how the role-players are briefed, how the examiners make their assessments is all useful and reassuring. But it is through their realistic approach to the practice cases, including filmed discussion and feedback, that the authors firmly establish their credibility as trustworthy guides to that career milestone that the CSA undoubtedly is. I would go further and suggest that, read throughout the training year and revisited periodically after it, their book is as much a guide to ordinary practice as it is to the exam.

In fact, I have only one critical comment to make. I think it should be retitled *How to Become a Good GP, and, Incidentally, Pass the CSA Exam.*

Bedmond, Hertfordshire
March 2014

Introduction

If you are preparing to take the RCGP Clinical Skills Assessment (CSA) exam, we have created this book and DVD for you. We are all experienced GP educators, we have worked with countless GP trainees, and we have lots of practical experience in helping them prepare for and pass the CSA. This book is based on our experience, as well as the experiences of GP trainees (we'll call them ST3s for consistency) who have recently sat the exam:

'My name is Shaleen and I passed the CSA quite recently. When I first started preparing for the CSA I felt daunted, to be honest – it seemed like such a lot to cover. But what really helped me was practising real cases in small groups, with regular breaks, and sometimes just focusing on one skill at a time.'

The CSA is an exam about real-life general practice, based on the kinds of patients we all see every day in our surgeries. It is not designed to catch you out. It's OK to feel a little daunted when you begin to prepare for this exam – most of our ST3s feel like that. But if you see lots of patients, practise cases regularly and understand the key areas in which you are likely to be assessed, then there is no reason you shouldn't pass this exam.

The book has two main sections. The first part covers the **CSA exam** itself: how it is organised, what the examiners are looking for and what you can expect on the day. It also outlines the skills you need to develop to pass the exam, as well as common themes for failure. Throughout this we will be drawing on our own experiences as GP educators and the experiences of our ST3s who have recently taken the CSA and survived.

'My name is Mydhili and I passed the exam in 2010. I enjoyed a lot of my preparation; it was hard work but worth every moment. I found it helpful to remember that ultimately the CSA is trying to test what a normal GP would be expected to do in a normal clinic session.'

'My name is Sam and I passed the CSA last year. It was definitely worth starting to prepare nice and early. I also found that what really helped me was getting feedback on my own video-ed consultations, and practising cases with a group of colleagues.'

The second section of the book contains 36 **CSA practice cases** (that's 3 circuits of 13 cases). Clearly, they are not genuine CSA cases and any overlap with real cases is coincidental. Nevertheless, we have carefully chosen these scenarios to test the areas in which you may be assessed in the CSA exam. You can use them to practise in your revision groups during your CSA preparation, in a more formal tutorial group, or to read through on your own in conjunction with the DVD that we have also included to offer you some practical demonstrations.

The DVD includes 12 of the practice cases from the book, letting you see how colleagues tackle the consultations and hear our detailed feedback to the ST3s on their performance. We focus on the core skills that you need to demonstrate to pass the exam. Throughout the text in the book, you will find links to the relevant DVD cases to help you dip in and out. You can also watch a half-hour discussion between three recent ST3s who've passed the exam and an ST3 who's about to take it, offering their practical tips.

It may seem a remote prospect right now, but we hope that you will enjoy reading this book and preparing for your CSA. It may be an exam, but it's all about being a good GP. We think that the skills you learn while preparing for it are important and will stay with you throughout your career in general practice.

Finally, we'd like to wish you good luck in your preparation, and of course the very best of luck on the day. We'd also love to hear your feedback about this book so that we can make it even better for the next edition.

Raj Nair
Imtiaz Ahmad
Martin Block
Graham Easton

1 The CSA Exam

What is it, what are the examiners looking for and what can you expect on the day?

What is the CSA?

The RCGP website describes the CSA (Clinical Skills Assessment) as:

"an assessment of a doctor's ability to integrate and apply appropriate clinical, professional, communication and practical skills in general practice."

It goes on to say that the CSA is designed to (1):

"test a doctor's abilities to gather information and apply learned understanding of disease processes and person-centred care appropriately in a standardised context, making evidence-based decisions, and communicating effectively with patients and colleagues. Being able to integrate these skills effectively is a key element of this assessment."

There are three key messages to take from these statements:

1 The exam focuses on being patient centred.
2 Candidates need to make evidence-based management plans, in keeping with current UK general practice.
3 Candidates need to communicate using recognised communication techniques.

The second point acknowledges that recent knowledge of guidelines is helpful, so attempting the Applied Knowledge Test (AKT) in the same academic year as the CSA can be useful.

[Shaleen: I definitely felt more confident about being up to date with current guidelines having sat the AKT a few months before.]

Though we would not suggest relearning all the NICE guidelines, being familiar with the management of common conditions is definitely a bonus.

How to Pass the CSA Exam, First Edition. Imtiaz Ahmad, Raj Nair, Martin Block and Graham Easton.
© 2015 John Wiley & Sons, Ltd. Published 2015 by John Wiley & Sons, Ltd.

The CSA format

You can think of the CSA as a simulated typical morning surgery, seeing 13 patients in 10-minute consultations.

[Mydhili: It is a fair exam and supposed to test normal skills. Approach it like a morning surgery.]

The RCGP describes the format in this way (1):

"The CSA is a high-fidelity skills assessment based largely on the familiar and well-proven OSCE format providing an external, objective assessment of clinical skills at a standardised, pre-determined level of challenge. The validity of the CSA resides in its realistic simulation of real-life consultations. Patients are played by trained and calibrated role-players, and cases that are written and assessed by working GPs. Each candidate is allocated a consulting room and has 13 ten minute consultations."

The CSA covers a multitude of topics within medicine; in fact, it could include just about anything. And even within this vast range of potential topics, a station could test many more skills than merely history-taking and management. The format of the assessment allows for systematic sampling from the RCGP curriculum, using a selection blueprint as in Table 1.1.

To get a flavour of the range of clinical problems that the exam could cover, and which aspect of the consultation it could focus on, imagine filling out Table 1.2 with some examples. It will help you come up with possible cases too (we have used this sort of grid to choose our

Table 1.1 Skills and attitudes that could be tested in the CSA

Blueprint area	Descriptor
Data gathering and interpretation	Gathering of data for clinical judgement, choice of examination, investigations and their interpretations
Management	Recognition and management of common medical conditions in primary care. Demonstrates flexible and structured approach to decision-making
Co-morbidity and health promotion	Demonstrating ability to deal with multiple complaints and co-morbidity and to promote positive approach to health
Person-centred approach	Use of recognised communication techniques that enhance understanding of a patient's illness and promote a shared approach to managing problems
Professional attitude	Practising ethically with respect for equality and diversity in line with accepted codes of professional conduct
Technical skills	Demonstrating proficiency in performing physical examinations and using diagnostic and therapeutic instruments

Source: RCGP: CSA blueprint derived from the RCGP curriculum (2).

Table 1.2 Clinical case topics that could be tested in the CSA

Clinical Skills Assessment Case Selection Blueprint	Primary nature of case						
Primary system or area of disease ↓	Acute Illness	Chronic Illness	Undifferentiated Illness	Psycho-Social	Preventive/ lifestyle	Other
Cardiovascular						
Respiratory						
Neurological/Psychiatric						
Musculoskeletal						
Endocrine/Oncological						
Eye/ENT/Skin						
Men/Women/Sexual Health						
Renal/Urological						
Gastrointestinal						
Infectious diseases						
ETC						

practice cases – see Chapters 6 and 7). Don't be daunted – there's obviously a lot to cover here, but your ST3 year should prepare you for most of the typical cases, and with a little practice and a systematic approach (which we will outline later), you should be able to tackle the less familiar problems competently.

The marking schedule

So how do you pass? What are the examiners looking for?

Each case is marked in three domains (we will use the same colour codes that the RCGP uses in its document *Generic Indicators for Targeted Assessment Domains*):

- Data gathering, technical and assessment skills
- Clinical management skills
- Interpersonal skills

Each domain contains several positive and negative indicators- specific areas that the examiners are looking out for. These are outlined in Figure 1.1.

Each domain has four grades awardable:

- Clear pass (scores 3)
- Marginal pass (scores 2)
- Marginal fail (scores 1)
- Clear fail (scores 0)

So you can see that the maximum score per station is 9 (three clear passes across all three domains). The most important thing to remember about how you are marked is that **all three domains have equal weighting**. Therefore, if you run

out of time and do not spend a proportional amount of time on clinical management, you cannot score well. It is worth keeping an eye on a clock or stopwatch and when you reach around seven minutes, consider moving on to management. This will allow you time to ensure that you are sharing your management plan, summarising appropriately and safety-netting (see Chapter 2 on consultation skills).

We would recommend doing this even at the expense of not doing as well in data gathering, as **you can only score a maximum of 3 in each domain**. So imagine that you have already scored 2 in the data gathering domain. By moving on you will sacrifice the final mark in that domain; but it should then be easier to score a couple of quick marks in the management domain. This is better than spending extra time on data gathering, only to gain the one extra mark possible, but nothing at all on management. It is also well worth looking at the feedback statements that the college publishes on areas where candidates trip up (3).

How the pass mark is set

Given that the maximum mark per station is 9, and there are 13 stations, the exam is marked out of a total of 117 (13 x 9). In general over the last few years, the mark needed to pass is around the high 60s. So, as a rough guide, scoring 70 should mean that you pass the exam. As you can see, this would mean scoring an

GENERIC INDICATORS FOR TARGETED ASSESSMENT DOMAINS

1. DATA-GATHERING, TECHNICAL & ASSESSMENT SKILLS: *Gathering & using data for clinical judgement, choice of examination, investigations & their interpretation. Demonstrating proficiency in performing physical examinations & using diagnostic and therapeutic instruments*

(Blueprint: Problem-solving skills, Technical Skills)

Positive Indicators	Negative Indicators
• Clarifies the problem & nature of decision required	• Makes immediate assumptions about the problem
• Uses an incremental approach, using time and accepting uncertainty	• Intervenes rather than using appropriate expectant management
• Gathers information from history taking, examination and investigation in a systematic and efficient manner.	• Is disorganised/unsystematic in gathering information
• Is appropriately selective in the choice of enquiries, examinations & investigations	• Data gathering does not appear to be guided by the probabilities of disease.
• Identifies abnormal findings or results & makes appropriate interpretations	• Fails to identify abnormal data or correctly interpret them
• Uses instruments appropriately & fluently	• Appears unsure of how to operate/use instruments
• When using instruments or conducting physical examinations, performs actions in a rational sequence	• Appears disorganised/unsystematic in the application of the instruments or the conduct of physical examinations

2. CLINICAL MANAGEMENT SKILLS: *Recognition & management of common medical conditions in primary care. Demonstrating astructured & flexible approach to decision-making. Demonstrating the ability to deal with multiple complaints and co-morbidity. Demonstrating the ability to promote a positive approach to health*

(Blueprint: Primary Care Management, Comprehensive approach)

Positive Indicators	Negative Indicators
• Recognises presentations of common physical, psychological & social problems.	• Fails to consider common conditions in the differential diagnosis
• Makes plans that reflect the natural history of common problems	• Does not suggest how the problem might develop or resolve
• Offers appropriate and feasible management options	• Fails to make the patient aware of relative risks of different approaches
• Management approaches reflect an appropriate assessment of risk	• Decisions on whether/what to prescribe are inappropriate or idiosyncratic.
• Makes appropriate prescribing decisions	• Decisions on whether & where to refer are inappropriate.
• Refers appropriately & co-ordinates care with other healthcare professionals	• Follow-up arrangements are absent or disjointed
• Manages risk effectively, safety-netting appropriately	• Fails to take account of related issues or of co-morbidity
• Simultaneously manages multiple health problems, both acute & chronic	• Unable to construct a problem list and prioritise
• Encourages improvement, rehabilitation, and, where appropriate, recovery.	• Unable to enhance patient's health perceptions and coping strategies
• Encourages the patient to participate in appropriate health promotion and disease prevention strategies	

Figure 1.1 Generic Indicators for Targeted Assessment Domains. Reproduced with kind permission of RCGP.

3. INTERPERSONAL SKILLS: *Demonstrating the use of recognised communication techniques to gain understanding of the patient's illness experience and develop a shared approach to managing problems. Practising ethically with respect for equality & diversity issues, in line with the accepted codes of professional conduct.*

(Blueprint: Person-Centred Approach, Attitudinal Aspects)

Positive Indicators	Negative Indicators
• Explores patient's agenda, health beliefs & preferences.	• Does not inquire sufficiently about the patient's perspective / health understanding.
• Appears alert to verbal and non-verbal cues.	• Pays insufficient attention to the patient's verbal and nonverbal communication.
• Explores the impact of the illness on the patient's life	• Fails to explore how the patient's life is affected by the problem.
• Elicits psychological & social information to place the patient's problem in context	• Does not appreciate the impact of the patient's psychosocial context
• Works in partnership, finding common ground to develop a shared management plan	• Instructs the patient rather than seeking common ground
• Communicates risk effectively to patients	• Uses a rigid approach to consulting that fails to be sufficiently responsive to the patient's contribution
• Shows responsiveness to the patient's preferences, feelings and expectations	• Fails to empower the patient or encourage self-sufficiency
• Enhances patient autonomy	• Uses inappropriate (e.g. technical) language
• Provides explanations that are relevant and understandable to the patient	
• Responds to needs & concerns with interest & understanding	• Shows little visible interest/understanding, lacks warmth in voice/manner
• Has a positive attitude when dealing with problems, admits mistakes & shows commitment to improvement.	• Avoids taking responsibility for errors
• Backs own judgment appropriately	• Does not show sufficient respect for others.
• Demonstrates respect for others	• Inappropriately influences patient interaction through own views/values
• Does not allow own views/values to inappropriately influence dialogue	• Treats issues as problems rather than challenges
• Shows commitment to equality of care for all	• Displays inappropriate favour or prejudice
• Acts in an open, non-judgmental manner	• Is quick to judge
• Is cooperative & inclusive in approach	• Appears patronising or inappropriately paternalistic
• Conducts examinations with sensitivity for the patient's feelings, seeking consent where appropriate	• When conducting examinations, appears unprofessional and at risk of hurting or embarrassing the patient

Figure 1.1 (*Continued*)

average 5–6 marks per station. You can do very well in some stations and thereby compensate for stations in which you may not perform as well.

Exact details on how the pass mark is set are on the college website, but they're quite complex and it's probably not worth getting too bogged down in this (4). It's very unlikely to affect your performance on the day – you just need to score as highly as you can. But in case you are interested, we will try to explain it simply here.

Essentially, having scored the candidate, the examiner is then asked to make a separate judgement on how they felt the candidate performed overall in the station. Most of the time a 'pass' or 'fail' is fairly clear cut. However, sometimes candidates come into a 'borderline' category. Perhaps they seemed to be performing well, only to run out of time; or perhaps they came up with the correct management plan, but didn't involve the patient in the decision-making process. Being classified as borderline won't affect that individual candidate's score on that station or their overall result, but the average of all the borderline candidates' marks is used to set the pass mark for that station. The same is done across all 13 stations, which means that borderline case scores are added together to calculate an overall borderline CSA score. This will vary day to day because of small overall differences in the difficulty of the cases. A small statistical adjustment is then made to that overall borderline CSA score (increasing it slightly to err on the side of caution), which produces the pass mark for the entire exam for that day.

None of this affects your personal score – it is simply a way to set a fair pass mark based on how all the candidates perform and the difficulty of the cases on the day, as well as taking variation among examiners into account. We have heard of trainees trying to choose certain days when they predict weaker candidates may sit the exam, as the pass mark might in theory be lower on that day (theoretically weaker borderline candidates would set a lower pass mark than better-scoring borderline candidates). However, there are so many other variables, including the difficulty of the case, that we think this is a pointless exercise. In any event, it is very difficult to get the exact day or time you would like for the exam. To pass you simply need to do as well as you can in the exam, not worrying about how the pass mark is set. It is much more important to be aware of the marking scheme (as outlined above).

What you can expect on the day

You can expect to feel a bit nervous – that's normal. The key is to channel the adrenaline into useful energy that will help you perform at your best. If you have seen plenty of patients and practised some CSA cases, then you should be well prepared. It may go without saying, but do allow plenty of time to get to the examination centre,

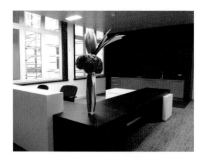
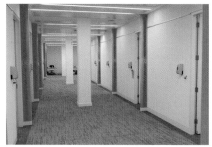
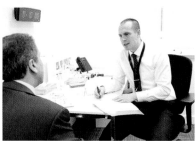

Figure 1.2 The RCGP exam centre and consultation room.

and make sure you've eaten something to keep you going. For guidance on what to wear, see the dress code (5).

[Shaleen: There is a 20-minute lecture-style briefing before the exam. They tell you how the day will run and how the iPads work.]

[Sam/Mydhili: Get there early. It's easy to find and don't worry, it's all fairly straight-forward on the day.]

Currently the exam consists of 13 live stations. You will be handed your pack of 13 patient histories before the start. This comes in the form of an electronic booklet on an iPad and each case is summarised at the front, although you need to turn to the actual page for more details. NB: There may be some more information overleaf, so don't forget to turn the page.

Don't worry if you have never used an iPad – it is very intuitive and there are marshals around to help you if you are really stuck.

[Shaleen: If you click on another case by accident during the exam, then the iPad flashes up a banner at the top telling you that the notes you are viewing do not relate to the current patient, so you don't have to worry about losing your place.]

There is a whiteboard next to the iPad for you to make notes and we would suggest you do so in case you forget something relevant in the consultation. The stations have been piloted and used many times and key information has usually been included for a reason, so it is worth highlighting pertinent parts (for example, a previous abnormal blood result or heavy smoking status). Be careful, though, that you don't focus too much on your own agenda or keep looking at the iPad or your notes instead of the patient.

You will have around 10 minutes before the start of the exam to read through your cases. There will be a short comfort break (of around 15 minutes) after seven cases, so you can finish reading the final cases then.

[Shaleen: I only read the first seven cases on the iPad in the initial 10 minutes so I could focus on these cases before the break.]

Tea and biscuits are provided during the break, but you may wish to bring an energy drink or chocolate bar with you to consume during the exam, which can be mentally draining. You should bring a doctor's bag with you containing the instruments that are listed (along with other essential information for candidates) on the college website (6). You cannot remove any material from the exam venue and you should not discuss cases that you have come across with anyone else. There is a clock in front of you that has a countdown feature. This can be helpful to keep track of time, but be

careful not to keep looking at it or put yourself under too much pressure. Your eyes should be making contact with the patient, not the iPad or the clock!

TIP: What CSA candidates can expect at the RCGP's new headquarters

Have a look at this short video from GP Online about what to expect on the day, including a glimpse behind the scenes into the preparation of examiners and role-playing patients, and a question-and-answer session that features detail about recent changes to the CSA.

http://www.gponline.com/Education/article/1184218/video-exclusive-csa-candidates-expect-rcgps-new-headquarters/

You stay in your doctor's room and the examiner and actor move along between cases. There is only one bell to start the station and one to finish. Each station lasts exactly ten minutes, with a two-minute break in between. Figure 1.3 summarises the rough structure of the exam.

Physical examinations

You will be expected to carry out some physical examinations. There are no 'real' physical signs to pick up, so practise doing focused examinations quickly (see Chapter 3 for what we recommend regarding common physical examinations) in around a minute.

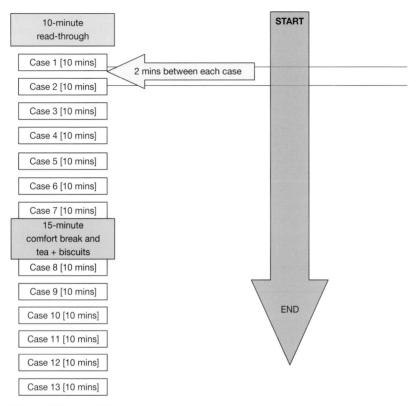

Figure 1.3 Structure of the exam.

Examples might be a focused chest exam or examining a joint.

Case A4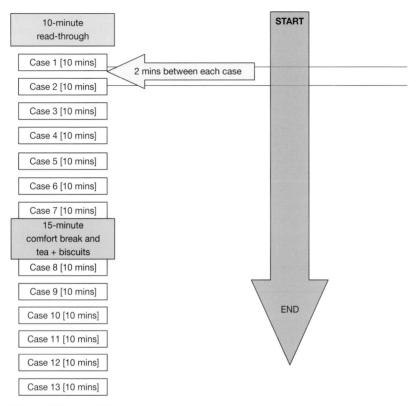

You should get up and attempt to examine the patient (remember to explain quickly to the patient what you would like to examine, and don't forget to ask for their permission and offer a chaperone if appropriate). Results from more intimate examinations or simulated physical signs (from, say, a 'normal' chest examination that you perform on a healthy actor) will be transferred to your iPad by the examiner. This is likely to be the only interaction you will have with the examiner, who sits out of your eyeline during the consultation.

Investigations

You may be expected to interpret simple investigations like ECGs, swab and blood results, as well as more complex investigations like spirometry results (not graphs). So it is worth spending some time reminding yourself how to recognise common primary care-related cardiac conditions such as atrial fibrillation or left ventricular hypertrophy, and what diagnostic criteria are needed to reach a diagnosis of asthma and COPD on spirometry. For a spirometry refresher, consider arranging a session with your practice respiratory nurse. You may need to demonstrate inhaler technique and peak flow meter readings too.

Home visits and telephone consultations

These types of scenario are increasingly common in the CSA, but not everyone will have a home visit or telephone consultation to tackle. Currently you will only be given one or the other, if at all. Although they are a little different to the usual stations, they tend to be more straightforward, partly because they are new – so there's no need to panic.

For the **telephone consultation** [Case B11], you stay in your room and use the telephone provided. The examiner and actor will be in a separate room connected to the telephone, listening to the consultation on loudspeaker. The scenario usually revolves around an out-of-hours call. Important things to remember here are:

1 Introduce yourself properly.
2 Establish who you are speaking to and that you have consent to give information (if relevant).

3 Do not forget the main marking domains of the CSA (see Chapter 3 on consultation skills): enquire about the psychosocial context of the problem, as well what the patient believes may be the problem, what may help and what they require.
4 If you are the out-of-hours GP, then you need to establish any past medical and drug history as well as allergies.
5 If you are recommending a visit to the out-of-hours base or the hospital, remember to enquire about transport and bear in mind the patient's social circumstances.
6 If a patient needs to be seen, try to get them to come to the base (if safe and appropriate) rather than wasting resources on a visit. However, if the patient cannot come and clearly needs to be seen, then you should arrange a visit as you would normally. Arguments with the patient are generally frowned on, so having a lower threshold for visiting is prudent!

Case B12

For **home visits**, you will be led to a separate room where there will be a new doctor's bag. The patient will be on a couch or sofa-bed and you should perform the consultation as you would normally, paying close attention to your surroundings and environment. The first five tenets above regarding telephone consultations are as relevant for home visits, especially bearing in mind the social context of the patient, and particularly when considering transferring the patient to hospital.

Some home visits can be quite complex (for example, a palliative care case as in Case B12). If you have not been caring for patients with these needs during your GP training, then it would be useful to spend a study session with the palliative care team. The communication skills required for these difficult end-of-life care conversations are often challenging and the more practice you have the better. Getting some feedback from your trainer or the palliative care nurses on how you discuss end-of-life care with a patient would be valuable, and a very good use of time both for the CSA and for real-life general practice. This experience doesn't only come regarding patients with advanced cancer – don't forget your house-bound heart failure and COPD patients, whom you may have seen before and whose end-of-life care needs tend to be overlooked.

[Sam: For a home visit, the marshal comes and you are taken over to a different room, perhaps with a couch or sofa. Try to pretend it's a real home visit.]

Paediatric cases

Nearly all candidates will have one paediatric case. This may or may not involve consulting with a child directly; the exam does sometimes use child role-play actors'. Of course, these children cannot be babies or small toddlers, so they are usually aged about 8, 9 or 10.

However, it will often involve consulting with a parent about a child who is not actually in the room. The paediatric stations are less likely to be an acute problem and more likely to cover more chronic issues such as constipation or difficult-to-treat eczema. Remember that if the child is not present, it may be appropriate to request a review appointment to see or examine the child (if relevant). In addition, the child's psychosocial context is paramount and it is essential to enquire about home and school as well as the usual developmental and social milestones. (Also see Chapter 5 on more complex cases.)

Prescribing

The issue of safe and appropriate prescribing is becoming increasingly important in the CSA exam. Within each circuit of 13 cases, it is likely that you will have several that involve some aspect of prescribing. You may well be asked to write out a prescription – this will be made very clear in the relevant station. While writing down the patient's correct details is obviously important (for example, their name and date of birth), you are not usually expected to write, for instance, the patient's entire home address.

When you are not specifically asked to write out a prescription, we would advise you to verbalise what you intend to write. For example, for a simple lower urinary tract infection (UTI), you could say: 'I would like to prescribe you an antibiotic called trimethoprim; you take one 200 mg tablet twice a day for three days.'

If you don't know a suitable drug or the correct dose, don't simply guess! Either check in your BNF (*British National Formulary*) or make it clear that you will need to verify the details of treatment. The examiners would much rather see a doctor who is comfortable admitting that he or she doesn't know something than one who bluffs their way in ignorance, putting the patient in danger.

[Shaleen: I put coloured tags (with no annotations) on sections in my BNF that I thought might be relevant so that I could find information easily if needed.]

When should I sit the CSA?

The answer depends on your personal circumstances and it is a good idea to discuss this with your trainer and programme director early in your ST3 year. As a general rule, you need to be comfortably seeing patients every 15 minutes in your usual surgeries. The exam consultations are timed at exactly 10 minutes, although you are not expected to do a comprehensive examination (see Chapter 3 about physical examinations) or write notes.

The CSA exam is now spread more evenly throughout the year, with sittings roughly monthly, so there is more flexibility in when you choose to take the exam. But in general, if you start your ST3 year in August, then attempting the exam the following February or March would be a reasonable plan. This would also give you a chance of sitting the exam again later on in your year, should things not go as well as hoped. However, if you or your educators are not confident with an attempt in February/March, then you are probably better off delaying your first attempt until later. There is very good evidence to suggest that your first attempt at CSA is your best attempt – if you have failed once, it may affect your confidence and overall ability to pass the exam. Don't try before you are ready.

If you are confident about passing early in the calendar year, the advantage of passing the AKT and CSA components of MRCGP is that you can concentrate on other non-examined, 'softer' aspects of the training year. We would strongly advise against sitting the CSA too early in the ST3 year, though, as consulting effectively within 15 minutes is a push for most trainees at the start of this year.

Summary

Just like any exam, the CSA is much more straightforward if you know what to expect and have prepared for it thoroughly. You can't predict which cases are likely to come up – it could be almost anything a GP might see. Nevertheless, understanding what the exam is trying to test, how it is run on the day and how the examiners use the marking scheme to assess you gives you a crucial advantage.

References

1. MRCGP Clinical Skills Assessment (CSA). RCGP website: http://www.rcgp.org.uk/gp-training-and-exams/mrcgp-exam-overview/mrcgp-clinical-skills-assessment-csa.aspx

2. RCGP GP Curriculum Overview. RCGP website: http://www.rcgp.org.uk/gp-training-and-exams/gp-curriculum-overview.aspx

3. General comments about features/behaviours observed in passing and failing candidates in the CSA. RCGP website: http://www.rcgp.org.uk/gp-training-and-exams/mrcgp-exam-overview/~/media/Files/GP-training-and-exams/General-comments-about-features-behaviours.ashx

4. MRCGP: The New CSA Standard-Setting System. RCGP website: http://www.rcgp.org.uk/gp-training-and-exams/mrcgp-exam-overview/~/media/Files/GP-training-and-exams/Standard-Setting-the-CSA-from-September-2010-onwards.ashx

5. Dress codes for postgraduate GP recruitment training and assessment. Royal College of General Practitioners/COPMED.http://www.rcgp.org.uk/gp-training-and-exams/mrcgp-exam-overview/~/media/Files/GP-training-and-exams/Dress-codes-for-post graduate-GP-recruitment-training-and-assessment.ashx

6. MRCGP Clinical Skills Assessment: Information for candidates. RCGP website: http://www.rcgp.org.uk/gp-training-and-exams/mrcgp-exam-overview/~/media/Files/GP-training-and-exams/CSA%20page/Microsoft%20Word%20-%2021%20%20CSA%20Information%20For%20Candidates%20v%2012%20MSSRKHTDJAC%20021013%20_2_.ashx

2 Consultation Skills for the CSA

A practical guide to consultation skills for the CSA exam

In this chapter we will cover:
- The three domains against which your consultation will be assessed in the CSA exam.
- A suggestion for how you might structure a consultation.
- Tips and techniques to make your CSA consultation effective.

The three domains

As we discussed in Chapter 1, your consultation in the CSA exam will be assessed against the three domains (colour coded here to reflect the colour coding of the RCGP Generic Indicators for Targeted Assessment Domains):
- Data gathering
- Clinical management
- Interpersonal skills

Your mark in each of these three areas will make up your overall mark for the station. These three domains should shape how you view the structure of the CSA consultation. Each domain contains several **indicators** – both positive and negative – to guide the examiners in their marking. We will highlight these indicators throughout this chapter like this:
- **Positive indicator:** Clarifies the problem and nature of decision required.

Our examiners' notes in the CSA practice cases (Chapter 7 in this book) also focus on these indicators in each of the three domains.

> ### TIP: Watch the time
> Manage the time you spend in your 10-minute CSA consultation on data gathering to allow enough time for clinical management.

It is vital that you familiarise yourself with the MRCGP 'Guide to how the CSA is marked'. This tells you what is expected of you in the CSA consultation and

How to Pass the CSA Exam, First Edition. Imtiaz Ahmad, Raj Nair, Martin Block and Graham Easton.
© 2015 John Wiley & Sons, Ltd. Published 2015 by John Wiley & Sons, Ltd.

outlines the Generic Indicators for Targeted Assessment Domains. It is available on the CSA section of the MRCGP website at this web address: http://www.rcgp.org.uk/gp-training-and-exams/mrcgp-exam-overview/~/media/Files/GP-training-and-exams/Guide-to-how-the-CSA-is-marked.ashx).

- **Read** this document.
- **Print it out** and refer to it when you are practising cases.

A structure for the CSA consultation

With the three CSA domains in mind, a typical consultation might have the broad structure shown in Figure 2.1.

Clearly, not every consultation will fit neatly into this structure, but it is helpful as a rough guide to thinking about how to tackle the CSA.

You have **10 minutes**. Think of your consultation as being split equally between data gathering and clinical

management. In reality you may spend a little longer on data gathering, but you should look to set aside about 4 minutes for management within a 10-minute consultation. Your interpersonal skills should be on show throughout the consultation.

We will look at data gathering and clinical management in turn, focusing on:

- Structure
- Key skills for data gathering and clinical management
- Key interpersonal skills in these domains

Data gathering

A typical structure for this part of the consultation would be as shown in Figure 2.2.

Introduction

This may sound obvious, but be warm and welcoming as you introduce yourself to the patient. First impressions really do count. Notice how your colleagues welcome their patient and begin the

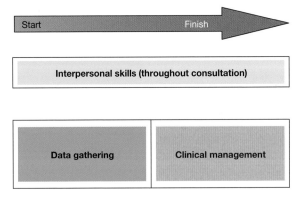

Figure 2.1 A broad structure for the consultation

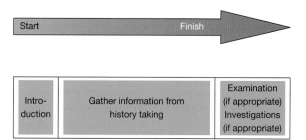

Figure 2.2 A typical structure for data-gathering

consultation. Think of people who have made **you** feel welcome – how did they achieve this? If you put the patient at ease, then they are more likely to be comfortable talking to you, and also more likely to offer you the information you need. The introduction is the part of the consultation that you can control and practise naturally in all the consultations you have during your ST3 year.

Consultation skills courses and books often talk about how a doctor should start a conversation. Neighbour (1) mentions keeping silent, and we often use power-sharing opening phrases such as '*What brings you here today*?' or '*What would you like to discuss today*?'. It's usually best to open with a phrase you normally use and one you find works for you with real patients. So if you normally start with the question '*How can I help you today*?', then keep doing that if it works for you. If you use phrases or techniques that you aren't familiar with and you haven't tested with real patients, then there is a danger that you will come across as artificial. If you don't sound

authentic, in the CSA consultation the actor's response to '*What brings you here today*?' might be '*My car*'.

Silence as an opening gambit from the doctor may not be the most practical use of time in the CSA, though it holds some merit in real-life general practice.

Gather information from history taking

The overall aim of this part of the consultation is to identify and clarify the problem that the patient has brought to you. This is the foundation of your consultation.

• **Positive indicator:** Clarifies the problem and nature of decision required.

It is important to **allow the patient time at the beginning to express why they have come to see you**.

The patient will often have a clear idea why they have come to see the doctor. They've probably been rehearsing this on their way to see you. Don't interrupt them at the beginning until they have had a chance to say their piece. The evidence suggests that this will usually take no more than a minute or so. Think of it as the '**golden minute**' (Figure 2.3).

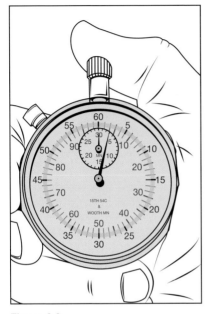

Figure 2.3

Respond with questions to explore further. Responding appropriately can be challenging in an exam situation, especially when you are feeling nervous and under time pressure. If a patient mentions a cue that suggests there is more to explore, try to respond as you would normally.

This should enable you to fulfill the following:

- **Positive indicator:** Identifies and clarifies the **patient's problem**.
- **Positive indicator:** Explores the patient's **agenda, health beliefs and preferences.**

Remember, this part of the consultation should flow naturally, just like your consultations in general practice. Here is an example:

TIP: Use videos

Watch a video of yourself consulting. Note when you ask your first question. Ask yourself whether you think the patient has said what they wanted to say by this point.

Listen and respond

Listen to what the patient is telling you. Show the patient that you are listening: use silence appropriately, as well as active listening with good eye contact, open body language and appropriate nodding. Paralanguage such as 'Mmm', 'OK' and 'right' can also be useful, but you need to do this naturally.

PATIENT: *'I've been feeling down for weeks now, but I haven't told anyone. I keep crying all the time and forgetting stuff, and there's not a day goes by that I don't wish that I didn't have this baby.'*

DOCTOR: 'That must be terrible.'

PATIENT: *'It's really awful, I've never felt as bad as this in my life. I just don't know what to do, I really don't.'*

DOCTOR: [Silence, with encouraging non-verbal communication (e.g. nodding) for a few moments, then patient continues.]

PATIENT: *'I was thinking, maybe I'm depressed, but I've never been depressed before so I don't know what that means or anything…'*

By giving the patient time and space to tell their story, you often save a lot of time and trouble later on.

Two tips we recommend as you progress:

1 Move from **open questions** to **closed questions**.

2 Be alert to **cues**.

- **Positive indicator:** Appears alert to verbal and non-verbal cues.

Move from open questions to closed questions

Open questions allow you to explore the problem, gain a better understanding of the patient's health beliefs and in this way open up the consultation. They will lead you to learn much more about the patient's problem and their agenda. Here are some examples of open questions:

- *'Tell me more about the pain.'*
- *'What does depression mean to you?'*
- *'Anything else you've noticed, apart from the diarrhoea?'*

Closed questions should generally be used after your open questions. They should be relevant and focus on:

- Filling the gaps and clarifying the details (in your understanding of the problem or the patient's agenda).
- Ruling out red flags.

It can feel quite jarring for the patient as you move from encouraging, open questions to more targeted and business-like closed questions. It can be helpful to **signpost** this change of direction clearly (Figure 2.4). For example:

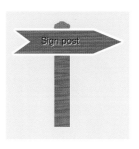

Figure 2.4

- *'I just need to ask some more focused questions now, if that's OK?'*

Here are two example interactions using closed questions:

> DOCTOR: 'So let me just clear a few things up. How has your sleeping been?'
>
> PATIENT: *'Terrible, I sleep for about a couple of hours and that's it. Then I'm exhausted the following day.'*
>
> DOCTOR: 'That must be tiring. How about your appetite?'
>
> PATIENT: *'To tell you the truth, I've been comfort eating.'*
>
> **Or**
>
> DOCTOR: 'Tell me, has there been any blood with this diarrhoea?'
>
> PATIENT: *'None that I've noticed.'*
>
> DOCTOR: 'What about weight loss?'
>
> PATIENT: *'Again, nothing I've noticed, but I don't tend to weigh myself.'*

With your closed questions it is important that you cover ground that is **relevant** to the patient's problem and that you stay

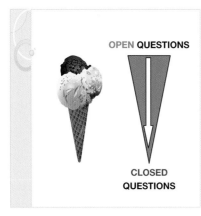

OPEN QUESTIONS

CLOSED QUESTIONS

Figure 2.5

focused. Don't repeat yourself and don't go over ground that you have covered already. Be efficient in your closed questions.

- **Positive indicator:** Gathers information from history taking in a systematic or efficient manner.

You could think of moving from open to closed questions as starting broadly and then narrowing down, like a cone (Figure 2.5).

Red flags
Case B2 📹

Closed questions are very useful for ruling out red flags – and showing the examiners that you are safe and understand the potentially serious problems that you don't want to miss in a presentation. In some situations it's obvious that you need to ask about red flags: for example, in a 60-year-old man with a recent change in bowel habit, you

would also ask about rectal bleeding, weight loss and appetite. But don't forget the less obvious cases: for example, an upper respiratory tract infection in a former smoker. In this case you might quickly check about weight loss, night sweats, haemoptysis, chest pain, foreign travel or exposure to tuberculosis.

Be alert to cues
Case A12 📹

We would strongly encourage you to keep your eyes and ears open to cues. These can often be the gateway to the patient's agenda, health beliefs and preferences. Be alert to them and respond to them. Here are a couple of examples where the doctor is alert to cues, and picks up on them:

> PATIENT: *'I've been spending a lot of time at home and I've been having some pretty dark thoughts.'*
> DOCTOR: 'Dark thoughts? Are you OK to talk about these?'
> **Or**
> PATIENT: *'I guess I would have expected the diarrhoea to settle down by now, but it hasn't, and you never know about these things…'*
> DOCTOR: 'OK…' [allows a moment of silence and some encouraging body language].
> PATIENT: *'Yeah, I remember my uncle had bowel cancer, and he started out with diarrhoea.'*

Watching videos of your consultations is a great way to learn more about cues. Look out for the ones you pick up and the ones you miss. We have highlighted several cues (verbal and non-verbal) in the DVD accompanying this book.

Psychosocial issues

Be alert to the psychosocial aspect of the consultation. The patient may give you cues, or you may have to ask more directly, but placing the illness in the context of the patient, their family and those around them is paramount. The same illness can affect different patients in very different ways. It is important to be appropriately curious about what is happening in the patient's life and how their illness or problem is affecting them in their day-to-day life.

• **Positive indicator:** Elicits psychological and social information to place the patient's problem in context.

Who else lives with the patient and how are the relationships between them and their partner? Are they in work and if so, what do they do? Is their illness affecting their work or vice versa? Showing some empathy to the social difficulties they are having would be a good way to form rapport. Is their problem affecting hobbies, or sport perhaps?

If their problem is a long-term one and they are presenting for the first time, often it is worth enquiring why they are coming to see the doctor today. Has something happened recently that makes them visit the doctor now?

TIP: Use summarising
Case A11 ▣

Summarising isn't only something you do at the end of the consultation. It can also be really useful as you move towards the closing exchanges in your data gathering. This is an idea that Roger Neighbour develops in his book *The Inner Consultation* (1). It is an effective way to check in with the patient and to clarify your own thoughts before moving on. Here's an example:

Doctor: 'So from what I understand, you've been coughing for a month now, and you're thinking that you have an infection that might need some antibiotics.'
Patient: *'Yes, that's right.'*
Doctor: 'OK, good. I'd like to examine you know, if that's OK.'

TIP: Don't use unnatural phrases to explore agenda and impact

• **Positive indicator:** Explores patient's agenda, health beliefs and preferences.
• **Positive indicator:** Explores the impact of illness on patient's life.

The RCGP examiners have highlighted in their feedback that weaker candidates will use stock phrases that seem unnatural in their data gathering. It is important that you explore the patient's agenda, health beliefs and preferences, and the impact of the illness on their life, but you should try to elicit these **naturally** during your data gathering, by **listening and responding to the patient** and being **alert to cues.**

If the impact or agenda has not become apparent during your data gathering, then some specific questions may be necessary **later**: for example, '*What impact is this having on your life*' or '*How is this affecting you*?'.

Examination

To complete your data gathering it is often appropriate to proceed to a physical **examination**. If this is what you would do in real-life general practice, then you should communicate this **to the patient**. This important part of the consultation is considered specifically in Chapter 3.

Explanation

You can think of the explanation stage in the consultation as the bridge between data gathering and clinical management (Figure 2.6).

The **explanation** is a pivotal point in the CSA consultation. It is when you make sense of your data gathering before going on to your clinical management.

- **Positive Indicator:** Provides explanations that are relevant and understandable to the patient.

When you are explaining anything to the patient you should try to use clear language, avoiding unnecessary medical jargon and drawing on the patient's own understanding of the problem.

Use clear language free from medical jargon

You are likely to lose marks if you use too much complicated medical jargon when talking with patients, as shown in Figure 2.7.

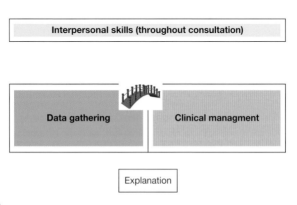

Figure 2.6

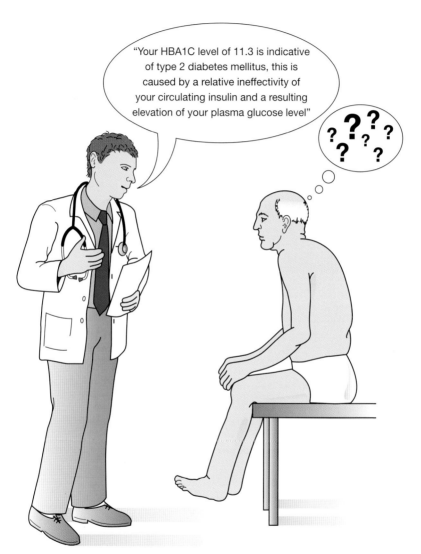

Figure 2.7 The dangers of using medical jargon

The patient would be much less bemused if the doctor used much less jargon, used clear language, and checked that the patient understood. For example:

> DOCTOR: 'Your blood test shows that you have diabetes. Do you know anything about diabetes?'
>
> PATIENT: *'My dad had diabetes – that's where you get high sugar, isn't it?'*
>
> DOCTOR: 'That's correct. The body's own way of controlling sugar stops working well, which means that the sugar level in the blood rises. This can lead to problems.'

Draw on the patient's understanding and health beliefs
Case A3

We all try to make sense of life in terms of what we already know or understand about it. So explanations tend to be more effective if they refer in some way to the patient's own existing understanding of the problem. Some candidates' explanations to a patient with chest pain might go something like this:

Doctor: 'This pain you're getting is most likely to be coming from your ribs…'

Stronger candidates might say something like this:

Doctor: 'You told me that you thought the pain in your chest might be coming from your heart. But having asked further questions and examined you, I think that's extremely unlikely. I think I can reassure you that the pain seems to be coming from your ribs.'

Here's another example of incorporating the patient's beliefs into your explanations:

Doctor: 'I'm sure you're right. Having assessed you, it does seem that all the difficulties you've been having with your relationship and your job have led to you becoming depressed.'

Here's another example – even with a straightforward problem like a sore throat, it's still worth exploring the patient's beliefs and trying to incorporate them into your explanations.

> DOCTOR: 'How can I help?'
>
> PATIENT: *'I've had this sore throat for a few days.'*
>
> *A few exchanges follow, exploring how it affects the patient; red flag symptoms and differentials.*
>
> DOCTOR: 'Have you had a problem like this before?'
>
> PATIENT: *'Yes, last time I left it for a while and didn't come to the*

*doctors, and in the end I got really
sick and needed to go to hospital
for a drip of antibiotics.'*

DOCTOR: 'What were you told was
the diagnosis last time?'

PATIENT: *'Oh, tonsillitis. It was very bad.'*

DOCTOR: 'So can I clarify, last time things
were left too long and you ended up
needing hospital treatment and were
quite sick. We want to avoid that?'

PATIENT: *'Yes.'*

*The doctor then examines the patient
and is happy that the patient does
not meet the Centor criteria (a set of
criteria that may be used to identify
the likelihood of a bacterial infection
in patients complaining of a sore
throat* (2)).

DOCTOR: 'I have examined you and
listened to what you have told me
and am pleased to tell you that
your sore throat is different from
the one you had last time. From
what you told me, it sounds like
last time you had a severe bacterial
infection that quite rightly needed
antibiotics. However, on this occasion there are no signs of a bacterial infection: you don't have a
temperature and there is no pus on
your tonsils, thankfully. This means
it is a different illness and is likely to
be a viral illness, which will not
respond to antibiotics but should
not get as bad as last time and
make you more sick.'

In that example, the doctor would not
have been able to incorporate the
patient's heath beliefs so effectively into
his explanation had he not already
explored them. Always try to take account
of patients' health beliefs if you can.

Exercise: Explanations

You could practise giving explanations in pairs, role playing a doctor
and a patient. Here are some topic
suggestions:

- A diagnosis of **type 2 diabetes**
  in someone who has told you
  that this condition 'runs in the family' (both the parents have it, and
  their father is now on insulin).
- A diagnosis of **atrial fibrillation**
  in an elderly man who was worried that the palpitations he was
  experiencing were signs of a 'heart
  attack'.
- A diagnosis of **chlamydia** to an
  asymptomatic teenage girl who was
  told she should 'get tested for STIs'
  by a former partner.
- A diagnosis of **viral labyrynthitis** in
  an anxious man who is worried
  about a brain tumour.
- A referral for **colposcopy** in an
  asymptomatic woman with moderate
  changes noted on smear.
- A referral for a **CT scan of the
  chest** in a smoker who has a
  suspicious lesion noted on chest
  X-ray.

Having explained what you think is going on, in terms that make sense to the patient, you can now move on to the next phase of the consultation: your management.

Clinical management

Your approach to **clear explanation** should continue throughout this part of the consultation, drawing on the ideas we have highlighted above, and offering clear explanations of **treatment options** or **proposed investigation**.

A typical structure of this section of the consultation could be as shown in Figure 2.8.

TIP: Know your management options

It may sound obvious, but don't forget this aspect in your preparation. You should aim to feel confident in the current management of common and important conditions. The examiners won't be trying to trick you. The exam is about real-life general practice, the kind of things that you see in your work every day. But in the heat of an exam, it may help to have a system for remembering the range of management options. For example:

- Primary healthcare team (for example, nurses, community psychiatric nurse, health visitor)
- Self-help (for example, keeping a sleep diary or cognitive behavioural bibliotherapy)

- Lifestyle (for example, diet, smoking, alcohol and exercise)
- Medication (don't leap for the prescription pad without considering other options too)
- Use of time (for example, planned follow-up)
- Counselling or other talking therapies
- Referral to specialist

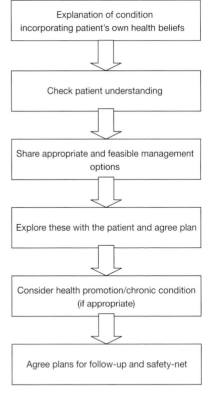

Figure 2.8 A typical structure for clinical management

Share appropriate and feasible management options
Case A2 ▢

This should begin with you deciding on appropriate management options for **the problem they have brought to you**.

To treat or not to treat

If not treating is a reasonable option, then let the patient know. For example:

> DOCTOR: 'As fungal infections of the toenail are not dangerous, we have the option of leaving this or offering you some kind of treatment.'
>
> DOCTOR: 'Now, as your thyroid test is borderline, we could treat you with some replacement hormones or we could keep an eye on you. Our decision here is often based on your level of symptoms, such as tiredness.'
>
> PATIENT: *'To be honest, I'd prefer to leave it for a bit. Could we see how we go and check in later in the year?'*

Sharing different treatment options

If you offer a choice between different treatment options, these should always reflect current best practice. This part is not about offering the patient whatever they want – it's more about 'putting on the table' what is **appropriate** and **feasible**.

- **Positive Indicator:** Offers appropriate and feasible management options.
- **Positive Indicator:** Makes plans that reflect the natural history of common problems.

For example:

> DOCTOR: 'There are a few things we can talk about that might be helpful in treating your depression. First, we could consider referring you for a talking therapy, such as counselling or cognitive behavioural therapy.'
>
> PATIENT: *'I had counselling 10 years ago when I was a student. It was really helpful and I'd be keen to have this again.'*
>
> DOCTOR: 'Yes, we can arrange for that. Another thing to consider would be an antidepressant medication. Do you know anything about those?'
>
> PATIENT: *'A little. Are they addictive?'*

Note that in this case the patient is not being offered one or the other – the doctor may decide to proceed with both talking therapy and medication. Do your best to offer balanced explanations of benefits and risks for each option:

- **Negative indicator:** Fails to make the patient aware of relative risks of different approaches.

It is also possible that you may want to explore other ideas for management later on in the consultation:

> DOCTOR: 'There are some other things we should talk about. For instance, we know that regular exercise can help in lifting depression. Any thoughts on this?'
>
> PATIENT: *I didn't know that. I used to quite enjoy swimming, but it's difficult to find time for this in a busy day, isn't it?*'
>
> DOCTOR: 'That's true.'
>
> PATIENT: '*But I know I should get back into it.*'

When sharing a management plan, you should **explain clearly** the **appropriate** management options, give the patient the **opportunity to participate** in this discussion and allow them to make the **final decision**.

- **Positive Indicator:** Works in partnership, finding common ground to develop a shared management plan.
- **Negative Indicator:** Instructs patient rather than seeking common ground.
- **Negative Indicator:** Appears patronising or inappropriately paternalistic.

Advising patient to pursue a particular treatment

Sometimes it's appropriate to advise a particular treatment. You may then need to explain and explore further as necessary. For example:

> DOCTOR: 'The rash that has spread over young Kia's skin is something called impetigo. This is caused by a bacteria that lives just under the skin. It's quite contagious. She may have caught it from one of her sisters or one of her friends at school.'
>
> PATIENT: '*OK, so what can we do about it?*'
>
> DOCTOR: 'I think she'll need some antibiotic medicine to clear this up.'

Advising a patient on a particular course of action may be crucial in acute emergency cases that you see in your CSA exam. Here's an obvious example:

Doctor: 'I'm concerned that you might be having a heart attack. I'm going to need to call for an ambulance. Is that OK?'

In these situations, the case is not about sharing management plans, but more about explaining the need for hospital assessment and treatment and dealing with psychosocial issues that may have an impact on this.

> **TIP: Don't offer inappropriate options**
> Your management should reflect current best practice. Consider this example of inappropriate management:

DOCTOR: 'You have a nasty cold. You could take some paracetamol, or I could give you some antibiotics. What would you like?'
- **Negative Indicator:** Decisions on whether/what to prescribe are inappropriate or idiosyncratic.

- Health promotion
- Management of associated chronic conditions

It won't be appropriate to do this in every consultation, but just like in your real-life work in the surgery, some encounters offer a good opportunity to tackle these areas.

Exercise: Management options (in pairs, role playing doctor and patient)

- Explain a new diagnosis of **cataract** in an elderly man who has just had an eye test and was told to discuss the results of this with the GP.
  Outline to the patient the two reasonable options: **surgery** and **not treating**.
- Explain a diagnosis of **tennis elbow** to a cleaner who is experiencing pain when she is working.
  Outline to her the possible treatment options, including **physiotherapy, steroid injection** and 'watching and waiting'.
- Explain to your healthy 18-year-old patient that you think her sudden onset of breathlessness and chest pain is potentially due to a **pneumothorax**. You would advise arranging an urgent **ambulance** to take her to A&E.

Exercise: Health promotion and managing chronic conditions

Think of (or practise) what you would say to the patient in these two examples:
- A postman in his 50s with a viral flare-up of **asthma.** After managing the patient's problem (by treating with a short course of oral steroids), you proceed to **offer health promotion** (smoking-cessation advice) and address his **chronic condition** (by booking him in to see the nurse for an asthma review – his control has been poor over the past six months).
- A 20-year-old man with a new diagnosis of **gonorrhoeal urethritis.** After managing the patient's problem (by treating with an oral antibiotic), you proceed to **offer health promotion** (on safe sex).

Health promotion and management of associated chronic conditions

Often, after managing the patient's problem, it is appropriate for you to consider:

In the CSA the strongest candidates will really bring the patient into this discussion, allowing them to be an active participant in the consideration of health promotion.

Health promotion does not always have to be done at the end of the consultation. If appropriate it can be discussed earlier – just bear in mind the time constraints of the consultation.

- **Positive Indicator:** Encourages patient to participate in appropriate health promotion and disease prevention strategies.
- **Positive Indicator:** Simultaneously manages multiple problems, acute and chronic.
- **Negative Indicator:** Fails to take account of related issues or of co-morbidity.

Follow-up and safety-net

As you start to think about closing the consultation, you need to consider:

- Follow-up
- Safety-net

Just as with your management, the key here is that what you do must be **appropriate**.

Follow-up

When would be an appropriate time to see the patient again? Allow the patient to be part of this discussion. Remember that the CSA exam should reflect your usual management – what a competent GP would do. Here are two examples of involving the patient in follow-up decisions:

> DOCTOR: 'I'd expect the antidepressants to start working in two to three weeks' time, so that might be quite a good time to come back and see me to see how things are going. What do you think?'

And

> DOCTOR: 'So, having started you on thyroxine, it is worth doing a blood test in around six to eight weeks to check your levels. How about you come and see me again a week or so after the test?'

Don't feel that you have to offer follow-up or review for the sake of it; sometimes an open door will suffice. Equally, it wouldn't be appropriate to agree to no follow-up, or even two months' follow-up, after starting antidepressants for the first time.

- **Negative Indicator:** Follow-up arrangements are absent or disjointed.

Safety-net
Case A3 📷

The idea of safety-netting – ensuring a contingency plan for the worst-case scenario – was first developed by Roger Neighbour in *The Inner Consultation* (1). The CSA guidance explicitly encourages appropriate safety-netting:

- **Positive Indicator:** Manages risk effectively, safety-netting appropriately.

When you need to safety-net (and this will not be in every consultation), the course of action must be **clearly expressed** and **appropriate.** It is really important to practise this skill in your groups or with your trainer. Ask yourself:

- What am I safety-netting for (what's the worst-case scenario)?
- What are the important signs that I need to communicate to the patient?

For example, in a patient with an asthma flare-up, you may arrange **follow-up** with the practice nurse for an asthma review, but you would also be keen to **safety-net** for a further deterioration in the patient's asthma:

> DOCTOR: 'So, as we agreed, the nurse is going to see you later in the month for your asthma review.'
>
> PATIENT: *'OK, doc.'*
>
> DOCTOR: 'So, I'd expect that things should start to improve within the next 48 hours. If things aren't improving after this, you should come back to see me here at the surgery. And if you find that things are getting worse – if you are starting to struggle with your breathing – then it's OK to call an ambulance straightaway.'

A thorough approach to safety-netting would include answering these questions:

- If your diagnosis is right, what **would you expect to happen**?
- How would you or the patient know **if you are wrong**?
- **What should the patient do then**?

For example, to a 56-year-old man who is having diarrhoea for seven days:

> DOCTOR: 'As I think this is a viral illness, I would expect the diarrhoea to settle down in the next week or so. However, if you're still not better by this time next month then it's worth coming back to see me, as I'll need to think about arranging some more tests.'

As with your follow-up, safety-net as you would do in real life, in real general practice.

Exercise: Safety-net

Think what you would do in these situations, or practise in pairs.

- How would you safety-net a depressed patient who you are following up in two to three weeks? Are there any specific considerations you would like them to be aware of?
- How would you safety-net a 5-year-old child with a viral upper respiratory tract infection over the last five days? What would you be worried about? How would you communicate this clearly?

Interpersonal skills

We have highlighted some of the key interpersonal skills as they apply to the data gathering or clinical management sections of the consultation. However, there are also overarching interpersonal skills that you should demonstrate throughout the consultation. These could be further divided into:

- Professionalism
- Patient-centredness
- Sensitivity/empathy

It is worth spending some time focusing on these areas specifically when practising the cases.

Professionalism

The examiners expect to see a professional doctor, who communicates values of moral integrity and respect for patients.

They expect you to be open and non-judgemental. This expectation on you is laid out explicitly within the positive indicators:

- **Positive Indicator:** Has a positive attitude when dealing with problems, admits mistakes and commits to improve.
- **Positive Indicator:** Demonstrates respect for others.
- **Positive Indicator:** Acts in an open, non-judgemental manner.
- **Positive Indicator:** Shows commitment to equality of care for all.
- **Positive Indicator:** Is cooperative and inclusive in approach.

Patient-centredness

You are expected to listen, communicate clearly and involve the patient in all decisions. The theme of patient-centredness runs throughout the interpersonal skills domain and can be further summarised by these positive indicators:

- **Positive Indicator:** Shows responsiveness to patient preferences, feelings and expectations.
- **Positive Indicator:** Enhances patient autonomy.
- **Positive Indicator:** Does not allow own views/values to inappropriately influence dialogue.

Sensitivity/empathy
Case A12 ▢

It goes without saying that you are expected to be sensitive and understanding throughout the consultation.

As important as anything else in the consultation, the examiners are expecting to see a **caring and compassionate** doctor who can empathise with their patients.

- **Positive Indicator:** Responds to needs and concerns with interest and understanding.
- **Positive Indicator:** Conducts examination with sensitivity for patient's feelings, seeking consent when appropriate.

And finally... flexibility

Remember that sometimes you will have a consultation that won't fit neatly into the plan we've outlined above. This is OK. Just as in real general practice, sometimes you have to be flexible.

An example of this might be a consultation about blood results, which the patient is keen to know before going into any detailed data gathering. In these cases you'll have to go along with the natural rhythm of the consultation, coming back to the data gathering when this is appropriate.

But hopefully, if you use this structure to think about your CSA consultations, you will be thinking in a similar way to the examiners.

The CSA marking criteria are informed by what is considered to be an effective GP consultation. This section summarises briefly some of the key literature on consultation skills

Neighbour, *The Inner Consultation* (1)

Neighbour talks about the five tasks in a consultation:

- **Connecting** with the patient.
- **Summarising** where we are.
- **Handing over** an agreed plan to the patient.
- **Safety-netting**.
- **Housekeeping** of yourself as a clinician.

The Inner Consultation is a rich exploration of the consultation and is recommended reading for all GP trainees.

Pendleton et al., *The Consultation* (3)

Pendleton observed GP consulting and listed what happens during a consultation. These observations are often used by trainees to help navigate the consultation. Pendleton defined the following tasks:

- Define reason for attendance.
- Consider other problems.
- Choose appropriate action.
- Share understanding.
- Involve patient in management.
- Use time and resources well.
- Establish and maintain the relationship.

Berne, Games People Play (4; see case C9 for further detail)

In his transactional analysis technique, Berne describes three states that the doctor or patient may adopt during a consultation:

- Parent
- Adult
- Child

A consultation may become dysfunctional if the patient adopts the parent or child role in a consultation. Often an adult–adult interaction is most productive.

Stott and Davis, 'The exceptional potential in each primary care consultation' (5)

Stott and Davis highlight the value of being proactive within a consultation, and defined four key areas:

- Management of the patient's presenting problem.
- Modification of help-seeking behaviours.
- Management of continuing problems.
- Opportunistic health promotion.

Charon, *Narrative Medicine* (6)

Over the last 10 years there has been much written on narrative medicine and the value of doctors being attentive to the patient's story. Rita Charon's book *Narrative Medicine: Honoring the Stories of Illness* is an excellent introduction. If you are an inquisitive trainee, it is well worth a read.

References

1. Neighbour, R. (2004) *The Inner Consultation*. 2nd rev. ed. Milton Keynes: Radcliffe Publishing.
2. Centor, R.M., Witherspoon, J.M., Dalton, H.P., Brody, C.E. & Link, K. (1981) The diagnosis of strep throat in adults in the emergency room. *Medical Decision Making*, 1 (3), 239–246. PMID 6763125.
3. Pendleton, D., Schofield, T., Tate, P. & Havelock, P. (1984) *The Consultation: An Approach to Learning and Teaching*. Oxford: Oxford University Press.
4. Berne, E. (2010) *Games People Play: The Psychology of Human Relationships*. Harmondsworth: Penguin.
5. Stott, N.C. & Davis, R.H. (1979) The exceptional potential in each primary care consultation. *Journal of the Royal College of General Practitioners*, 29 (201), 201–205.
6. Charon, R. (2008) *Narrative Medicine: Honoring the Stories of Illness*. Oxford: Oxford University Press.

3 Physical Examination for the CSA

Brief tips on physical examination in the CSA

The number of physical examination cases seems to have increased steadily since the early days of the CSA exam. Even though there are fewer marks for this than for the rest of the consultation, it makes many candidates disproportionately anxious. Perhaps as GPs we are generally more comfortable with our history-taking skills than our technical examination skills. But in fact we are very experienced in performing focused examinations and this part of the CSA should not hold any particular horrors.

The RCGP document 'Details of the CSA' highlights the requirement for candidates to perform 'appropriate fluent examinations'. The CSA blueprint area of Technical Skills describes 'demonstrating proficiency in performing physical examinations and using diagnostic and therapeutic instruments'.

[Shaleen: The RCGP's eGP learning resource has a really useful section of videos of physical examinations at a standard expected of a GP.]

It is usually a small part of each consultation, but the knock-on effect of a poor examination can affect some candidates considerably. It is important to appear relaxed and comfortable when performing routine examinations, and to show that you are familiar with key diagnostic or therapeutic instruments. In addition, you should interact appropriately with patients, asking permission to examine them, explaining what you would like to examine, and then confidently talking them through what you are doing.

[Shaleen: During my revision I found it useful to rehearse how I would explain the examination to a patient before requesting their permission.]

Choosing the appropriate examination is the first step. whole-system examinations

How to Pass the CSA Exam, First Edition. Imtiaz Ahmad, Raj Nair, Martin Block and Graham Easton.
© 2015 John Wiley & Sons, Ltd. Published 2015 by John Wiley & Sons, Ltd.

are nearly always inappropriate and time-wasting. So it is important to think about what is *really* necessary, which will be driven by the history and cues from the patient.

[Shaleen: It is really important not to spend too long on the examination as you might not get enough time for discussing management (where a lot of the marks are).]

Permission, consent and exposure

Once you have decided what examination you would like to do, you should explain briefly what you have in mind and ask the patient's permission to carry it out (just as you would in normal practice). You might say something like this:

Doctor: 'OK, I'd like to examine you now, if I may. I'd like to listen to your chest, take your temperature, and examine your throat. Would that be OK?'

If the patient gives consent to be examined, there is no need to ask the examiner's permission as well.

In many instances, after you ask to do an examination the examiner will supply you with full details of examination findings. Examples might include blood pressure, weight, urinalysis and intimate examinations such as breast, rectal and genitalia examinations. If you would have done an intimate examination in normal practice,

then say that's what you would like to do; and it's still good practice to request a chaperone appropriately.

Patients should be adequately exposed, with consent. Given that the patients in the CSA are simulated patients (actors), it would be highly unlikely that you would be expected to expose any intimate or sensitive areas.

The two-minute focused examination

You should be able to examine patients in a fluent, focused and confident manner. Marks for the examination will usually form only part of one of the three domains, so spending a great deal of time on this may be detrimental to your overall performance. As a general rule, you should spend no more than two minutes on any given examination.

The starting point of most examinations is a good general inspection and you will usually get a mark for this in most cases. Just as in a driving test, it's worth making sure that it is obvious to the examiner what you are doing. So make sure that it's clear that you are making a general inspection of the patient – just don't overdo it and make it look unnatural.

After a general inspection, you will need to do a focused examination, relevant to the system(s) in question. The next section is our guide to the additional elements of the examination by system, which should get you most of the marks available. Each case is individual, of course – these are general recommendations that you may have to tailor to fit the patient in front of you.

[Shaleen: In some cases I found that as I got up to perform an examination, the examiner stopped me and released the examination findings to my iPad.]

Focused examinations by system
Cardiovascular
- Pulse (rate, rhythm)
- Blood pressure (to offer, as it is usually given by examiner)
- Jugular venous pressure (JVP) assessment (with patient lying at approximately 45 degrees and the doctor palpating to see if the JVP is obliterated)
- Palpating for heave/thrill and apex beat
- Auscultation: heart sounds in more than one position, and lung bases
- Peripheral oedema (ankle and/or sacral)

Respiratory
- Respiratory rate
- Finger clubbing
- Cervical lymph nodes
- Palpation: chest expansion and percussion
- Auscultation: lungs (comparing both sides)
- Peak flow (if appropriate)
- Inhaler technique (if appropriate)

Abdomen
- Pulse (rate)
- Blood pressure
- Clubbing
- Supraclavicular lymph nodes

- Pallor, jaundice
- Palpation: pain/mass/peritonism/ascites
- Auscultation: bowel sounds
- Urine dipstick
- Pregnancy test
- Rectal examination (if appropriate; also offer a chaperone)

Neurology
Cranial nerves 2–12
- CN 2–4 – eyes: pupil equal and reactive to light/full range of movement/visual fields/visual acuity/fundoscopy
- CN 5–7 – facial muscles movement and sensation
- CN 8 – ears: Rinne's, Weber's, otoscope
- CN 9–11 – resisted shoulder shrug/neck movements
- CN 12 – tongue movements/deviation

Peripheral nerves
- Tone (passive movements)
- Power (grading out of 5)
- Sensation (check dermatomes)
- Coordination
- Reflexes

[Shaleen: If it is a diabetic foot examination, then it would be appropriate to use a monofilament (as you would in clinic).]

Thyroid
- Pulses (rate, rhythm)
- Tremor
- Nails
- Eyes (proptosis, exophthalmos)
- Reflexes (slow relaxing ankle reflexes)

- Palpating from behind
- Swallowing
- Tongue protrusion

Musculoskeletal

Same general principles for all joints:
- Observe: adequate exposure, obvious inspection, compare both sides
- Move:
  ◦ Active (asking patient to move through range)
  ◦ Passive (doctor moving joint through range)
  ◦ Resisted (comparing both sides)
- Palpate: think anatomy! Look at patient's face when palpating
- Special tests: specific for each joint (see below for common conditions and special tests)

Wrist

Carpal tunnel syndrome:
- Pressure on median nerve
- Pain and neurological symptoms
- Special tests: positive Phalen's/Tinel's tests
  De Quervain's tenosynovitis:
- Inflammation of abductor pollicis longus/ extensor pollicis brevis tendon sheaths
- Special test: positive Finklestein's test (thumb in palm of hand and ulnar deviation of wrist)
  Trigger finger:
- Enlargement of nodule within flexor tendon sheath

Elbow
- Lateral epicondylitis, 'tennis elbow'
- Lateral elbow pain
- Extending hand/wrist

- Gripping objects/turning handles
- Special test: positive Mill's test, pain on resisted wrist extension caused by faulty technique, small grip, increase in sport/ activity, weak forearm muscles

Shoulder

Rotator cuff injury:
- Impingement
- Rotator cuff muscles (supraspinatus, infraspinatus, teres minor, subscapularis), stabilise ball in socket
- Painful arc: pain on active and passive abduction between 60 and 120 degrees
- Special test: positive 'empty can' test (arm at 90 degrees abduction, thumbs pointing down, resisting upward movement of arms causes pain)
  Adhesive capsulitis
- Frozen shoulder'
- Distinct phases: 1) pain predominant; 2) stiffness predominant
- Reduced range of movement in all directions, especially external rotation

Ankle

Ankle sprain
- Inversion injury
- Lateral ligaments affected
- Pain on passive inversion and active eversion
- Tender on palpation lateral aspect of ankle
- Special test: positive anterior drawer test if lateral ligaments are torn

Plantar fasciitis
- Predisposing factors (increased activity/ weight/change in footwear)

- Worse ambulation and activity
- Tight calves
- Point tenderness medial aspect plantar fascia

Knee
- Tender on palpation tibial tuberosity (Osgood-Schlatter's disease in adolescents)
- Tender on palpation joint lines, either OA or meniscal damage
- Special tests:
  - Valgus/varus strain for medial/lateral collateral ligaments
  - Anterior drawer/Lachman's test for anterior cruciate ligament
  - Full, deep squat and 'duck-walk'/waddle test for meniscus

Back
- Simple backache
- Nerve root pain
- Straight leg raise
- Lower limb neurology including reflexes
- Red flags – aged < 20 or > 55, trauma, unwell, weight loss, cauda equina, inflammatory
- Yellow flags: work related

Eyes
- Inspection
- CN 2–4 – eyes: pupil equal and reactive to light/full range of movement/visual fields/visual acuity (Snellen chart)/fundoscopy

ENT
- Otoscopy
- Throat inspection
- Cervical lymphadenopathy
- Nose inspection (including nostrils if relevant for e.g. nasal polyps, deviated septum)

4 Common Themes Affecting CSA Performance

The pitfalls and how to avoid them

The RCGP has published feedback on candidate performance after every exam since the CSA started in 2007. Prior to that, it provided general feedback on candidate performance in both the video module and simulated surgery aspects of the MRCGP exam (1).

There are key themes for poor performance, which are common to all three models of assessment (video, simulated surgery and CSA). In this chapter we summarise them in an easy-to-remember format, along with some extra tips on exam technique and dealing with nerves.

We hope that this is useful both for trainees, to help them remember pitfalls in the exam, and for trainers to concentrate on during role play in tutorials and while observing real and video consultations.

Failing to admit that you don't know

Obviously, as a GP there are many things that you are expected to know. Nevertheless, the examiners don't expect you to know everything. They are practising GPs who understand that medicine is full of uncertainties and that no doctor can ever know everything about all possible conditions. So if you find yourself uncertain or unsure about something important, don't pretend that you have all the answers. Don't bluff. That can put patients at risk and doctors who don't know their limits will make the examiners feel uneasy.

Time management

This is perhaps the most frustrating way for candidates to perform poorly in their

How to Pass the CSA Exam, First Edition. Imtiaz Ahmad, Raj Nair, Martin Block and Graham Easton.
© 2015 John Wiley & Sons, Ltd. Published 2015 by John Wiley & Sons, Ltd.

Table 4.1 Summary of features/behaviours of failing candidates from RCGP (1).

General features	Poor use of time
	Uneasy with or unable to acknowledge own ignorance or uncertainty
	More scripted summary than checking understanding
	Unaware of personal space
Data gathering	Formulaic questioning which can become interrogative
	Repetitive questioning
	Sequence of questions does not make sense
Clinical management	Insufficient knowledge base, or ability to think of realistic and effective alternatives
	Fails to integrate and apply knowledge
	Puts off making clinical decisions or a clear diagnosis
	Doesn't appear to grasp the dilemma if there is one
Interpersonal skills	Doctor-centred/patient's concerns not addressed
	Patronising
	Unable to explain effectively – may be wrong or not tuned to patient
	Inappropriate use of terms
	Over patient-centred to the detriment of clinical outcome

Source: Reproduced with permission from the Royal College of General Practitioners.

exam. It is also often how 'good' candidates can fail the exam.

The most common mistake is not leaving enough time to finish off the consultation. This will inevitably affect the marks you receive for management. You should structure your consultations and avoid repeating yourself too much. This includes over-use of summarising and double-checking. Good general consulting skills involve not focusing on one area for too long and in too much detail. A common error is to search obsessively for a non-existent hidden agenda; this may lead you down a time-consuming and fruitless blind alley.

By the time of the examination candidates should have a feel for what 10 minutes is like without needing to look at their watches continuously, although there is a countdown clock in the room. Practice really is essential here, both during real consultations and in role plays.

[Shaleen: There may be a station in which you might finish early. If you are happy you have covered what you needed to, then it is fine to finish – you don't have to rehash everything to see if you have missed something.]

Don't feel under pressure to get real-life consultations down to 10 minutes. Most candidates are on 15-minute consultations at the stage at which they take their CSA. That's usually fine, because real-life consultations include computer data entry, multiple problems and more thorough examinations to elicit genuine clinical signs. If you do finish with time to spare in your real surgeries, use the time to reflect on the consultation or read up around any management issues of which you are unsure.

[Shaleen: I wouldn't recommend taking lots of study leave before the exam. I treated every case in clinic as a potential 10-minute CSA case in the lead-up to the exam. I added in a few catch-up slots to write notes up on the computer between patients.]

During practice with your trainers and study groups, always stop after 10 minutes exactly and never allow time-outs. Be honest with each other if time management is an issue. That way, by the time of the exam, you should be expecting to complete the majority of your CSA cases within 10 minutes; though not doing so does not necessarily mean you have failed that station or the exam as a whole.

There are some occasions when finishing too soon may also be a sign of a problem, often with the next section – the history.

History

Asking questions is central to taking a history, but you need to ask them in an appropriate way. Failing candidates often ask questions in a formulaic or insincere way ('What are your expectations?') and don't seem to have listened to earlier responses from the patient. They also seem to ask questions haphazardly,

without any logical structure, as if desperately trying to make sure that they don't forget anything.

Red flags

Spotting important differential diagnoses and excluding 'red flags' is an essential part of even the most straightforward consultations encountered in general practice. If you fail to recognise these in the CSA, the examiners are likely to wonder how safe you are as a GP and may fail you in the history-taking part of that consultation. Unfortunately, the time pressures of the CSA, coupled with exam nerves, mean that it's easy to rush your history taking and thus lose valuable marks.

For example, if a 60-year-old man presents with a cough, it is essential to find out the cough's nature, duration, associated systemic symptoms (shortness of breath, chest pain, fever, tiredness, night sweats, appetite, weight loss), haemoptysis and smoking history. Good candidates will also explore other less common differentials by checking for dyspeptic symptoms, recent foreign travel and occupational history.

The danger of covering red flags in precise detail at the start of the consultation is the well-recognised problem of using closed questions too early. Good candidates adopt a balanced approach with effective use of open questions either before or after their series of closed questions. Some also preface (signpost) the closed questions by saying something like:

Doctor: 'I need to ask some more direct questions now to make sure I haven't missed anything.'

Failing candidates often shift clunkily from routine medical questioning into intimate or personal questioning without signposting to the patient what is coming.

Cues

Another easy mistake is ignoring or not picking up on cues. You don't have to pick up on them immediately every time – you could refer back to them later in the consultation. Cues are often associated with psychosocial factors important to that patient.

If a patient mentions that their symptoms are affecting them at work, some candidates will ask more work-related questions straight away to get a picture of the patient and their problem. Others may choose to continue with other aspects of the consultation and then come back to the cue later: 'You mentioned work earlier – is the cough affecting how you deal with clients during meetings?' Either strategy can lead to effective consultations. However, the potential danger of leaving the cue until later is that there's a risk of forgetting to mention it again. All it takes is running out of time, or an unexpected change in the course of the consultation.

In the CSA the actors have often been primed to send cues, so it is important to listen carefully and also watch for non-verbal cues. Open questions followed by good consulting skills will usually pick out any important cues.

Establishing health beliefs

Perhaps the most important part of the history detail for the CSA is establishing a patient's health beliefs. Even though this is a core principle of Pendleton's consultation model [2], candidates do not generally perform it well. This is because it *is* difficult!

In the video consultations of the old MRCGP exam, candidates were effectively given the mark sheet beforehand and so knew exactly which areas they had to cover. This mark sheet was based on Pendleton's consultation model. Despite this, it was consistently the most poorly performed part of the old exam. One of the areas that was particularly poorly performed was establishing patients' health beliefs and subsequently taking account of these beliefs when creating a shared management plan.

The problem that candidates had was not a lack of trying to ask questions about health beliefs, but more a lack of **understanding** about what it means to establish a patient's health beliefs.

Poorer candidates often use formulaic questions such as '*What do you think has caused the problem?*' and think that they have covered this aspect. Patients (and actors in this case) can give a range of limited answers to this, such as '*I don't know*', '*You are the doctor*' or '*That's why I came to see you*'. It is obvious that further questioning will be needed. Even when patients respond with answers such as '*I think I have pneumonia*', further appropriate questions are still required truly to establish health beliefs: What is their understanding of pneumonia? Is it a minor respiratory infection? Is it something that definitely requires antibiotics? Does it mean hospitalisation, as happened to their great aunt a few years ago? Is it a precursor of cancer that their work colleague told them about? Does it require an urgent X-ray as they read on the internet?

Failing candidates tend not to explore health beliefs fully by asking those sorts of questions. You can now see what we need to take our questioning a step further, for example: 'It's interesting you have mentioned pneumonia, do you know much about it?'

Management

One of the three domains in the marking schedule is for clinical management. Any prescribing or referral is included in this domain. If candidates overrun their allotted time before discussing management, then it will usually result in a fail for that section of the station. Many poor candidates also over-run because they delay making a clear diagnosis or management plan, simply because their grasp of clinical management is not strong enough.

[Mydhili: I still ran over in two or three cases but passed them. If that happens don't panic – just carry on to the next case.]

[Sam There's no paperwork, no computer screen and no Quality and Outcomes Framework, so it's better than a real surgery!]

Good management has to be grounded in current best practice. We are continually reminded that the CSA is a test of communication skills, while the AKT (Applied Knowledge Test) has already tested our clinical knowledge. A range of clinical knowledge is, however, required for the CSA exam. This is why it is a good idea to do the CSA soon after passing your AKT, when your knowledge base will be high. If there is up-to-date national guidance, it is important not to ignore it during your management plan. It is also useful to remember that these are guidelines and in some CSA cases (as in real life) flexibility is required. Your negotiation skills will be tested, as will your use of common sense.

Be careful not to over-investigate or over-refer – you are being judged on what you would do in real-life general practice by examiners who are working GPs.

The key to formulating a management plan is to try to be patient-centred throughout your consultation, which extends to formulating a shared management plan with your informed patients. In general, failing candidates are more likely to adopt a doctor-centred, paternalistic approach to management plans. Reflecting on patients' ideas about their conditions and expectations for treatment can help avoid this. Offering management options is useful, but this needs to be done appropriately, especially with emergency cases. Failing candidates can also misinterpret patient-centredness as agreeing to anything the patient asks for – even when it could have a detrimental effect on clinical outcomes.

Finally, beware of vague follow-up plans and fuzzy safety-netting. Give your patient clear timeframes. For example: '*I would like to see you again in two weeks' time*.' When safety-netting, be *specific* about what you expect to happen if you are right about your diagnosis, and what to look out for if you are wrong and what the patient should do in that situation.

Explanation
Jargon
Most CSA cases involve common medical conditions encountered in general practice. However, when it comes to explaining a diagnosis or management plan, poor candidates often use complex medical jargon or pitch their explanation at a level the patient can't understand. And when the actor patient clearly shows that they don't understand (perhaps with a quizzical expression), the candidate simply ignores the cue and keeps going.

With the nerves of an important exam and the accompanying time pressures, even explaining simple conditions or procedures can be challenging. This is another area in which you can improve considerably with practice. There are a

number of ways of practising this: making lists from conditions you see every day, or taking turns to explain conditions in study groups or at home with your friends and family, and also in tutorials with your trainer.

Incorporating health beliefs
Another sign of a weaker candidate is not tailoring explanations to the patient's agenda or understanding. A useful tip is to incorporate your patient's health beliefs or agenda explicitly into your explanation. For example, if a patient strongly believes that his trigger finger is due to arthritis like his grandmother had, then you can suggest:

Doctor 'I can see why you have made a link between the two conditions. However, I disagree, as the cause is very different. You have thickness of the tendon in the palm of your hand that is causing a problem at the end of your finger. A tendon is the end of your muscle that attaches to your bone. It sounds as though your grandmother may have had wear and tear of the small joints in her hand, which is a common form of arthritis in old age. Fortunately, there is no link between the two conditions and yours should improve with the management options I will now discuss with you.'

A bad station
All of us have bad moments in clinical exams, but how we respond can affect the whole day. Try to think positively between stations and approach each

new station without any 'baggage' from the previous one. Focus on what went well (there are three domains, so even if you do not know the diagnosis, good interpersonal skills will score some points in communication at least and some for data gathering). It is worth remembering that examiners and actors want candidates to perform well, so approaching each new station with confidence is important.

[Shaleen: I found it useful during revision to do two cases back to back and then debrief at the end, as this replicated the stress of the exam to a degree (and helped me get used to doing and concentrating on another case straight after one that may not have gone so well).]

So if you do think you've had an awful station, it's vital to try to put it out of your mind. The exam tests your performance across all the stations, and the examiner at your next station won't have seen your previous disaster. So you can start with a blank sheet. And remember that you are allowed some 'less than ideal' stations while still reaching the pass mark. Keep calm and carry on.

[Sam: If you have a bad case, try to leave it behind and don't let it spill into the next one. They do come quickly. Try to be as fresh as possible for the next one.]

Exam nerves

Exams are always nerve-wracking, especially when they involve a live performance, as in the CSA. The examiners understand that – exam-day nerves are normal. What is important is that you use them to your advantage so that you are focused on the job in hand and feeling sharp.

It is worth mentioning that most trainees we know say that after the first case or two they generally forget that they are in an exam situation and start not to notice the examiners. Just focus on the patient – as you would in real life – and do your best. Real-life general practice can be messy, imperfect, stressful, fascinating, even enjoyable; you can expect the CSA exam to feel very similar!

References

1. General comments about features/ behaviours observed in passing and failing candidates in the CSA. RCGP website: http://www.rcgp.org.uk/gp-training-and-exams/mrcgp-exam-overview/~/media/Files/GP-training-and-exams/General-comments-about-features-behaviours.ashx
2. Pendleton, D., Schofield, T., Tate, P. & Havelock, P. (2003) *The Consultation: An Approach to Learning and Teaching.* Oxford: Oxford University Press.

5 Complex Cases in the CSA

Tips on some of the more challenging types
of CSA case

Just as in your morning surgery, some consultations in the CSA are more complex than others. These can be particular situations or types of patient that throw up special challenges. For example, your patient may have a disability that affects how you can communicate, they may be extremely angry, or perhaps you have to give them some difficult news. In this chapter we offer some tips on how to approach some of the more complex cases you may encounter:

- Disabled patients
- Elderly patients
- Paediatric patients
- Angry patients
- Demanding patients
- Language barriers
- Breaking bad news
- Health promotion

Disabled patients

The case notes should make it clear if a patient has a disability, so you should have a little time to gather your thoughts. You should consider what type of disability it is, and what you could do to make the consultation run more smoothly.

If the nature of the patient's disability isn't immediately clear, then try to establish early on in the consultation what type of disability is involved, how it might affect communication and what you could do to help. For example, a partially deaf patient may be able to lip read; you could help by turning towards them so that they can see your face fully and speaking very clearly (without coming across as patronising).

On the other hand, for a patient with severe deafness you may need to write things down. For a partially sighted person,

How to Pass the CSA Exam, First Edition. Imtiaz Ahmad, Raj Nair, Martin Block and Graham Easton.
© 2015 John Wiley & Sons, Ltd. Published 2015 by John Wiley & Sons, Ltd.

it would be thoughtful to ask if the light in the room is adequate for them, or if they would prefer written information. If written information, then does this need to be in Braille or large font or audio format?

Use your normal patient-friendly language and don't avoid words like 'see' or 'look' or talking about activities that involve sight (1). You should continue to face blind patients as you would normally and use non-verbal cues; these will help set the tone of your language, which will help in communication. Never assume that any disability necessarily means a lack of autonomy or understanding, though it is important to appreciate that those with a learning disability may be able to consent to some examinations and procedures but not to others. When you're looking after patients with disabilities, it is even more important to explore the social and psychological impact of the problem on the patient and their family.

With any examination, it's important to explain exactly what you are going to do before physically touching the patient. It is good practice to remind the patient that they can stop you at any point, verbally or otherwise (for example, waving a hand). You may be asked to guide a blind patient around the room; see the tip box for advice.

It can be hard to get experience with patients with a disability during your training, so it might be worth sitting down with your trainer and identifying suitable patients for you to consult with. This may be as part of an annual health check-up that some practices are advised to do, or going on a home visit with your trainer. Watching how they consult may also provide good learning material. It would be good to have an idea of the support and services available for specific common disabilities (such as talking books or visual aids).

Elderly patients

GPs are seeing more and more elderly patients, many of whom are fitter than our younger patients. Nevertheless, some elderly patients may have specific needs: for example, they may need you to take your time when explaining things or when asking questions. They may have a hearing or visual loss (see the section on disabled patients). Elderly actor patients (just like real patients) may not relish being examined multiple times in one day, so it's worth being understanding and gentle when you examine them.

If the patient has dementia, bear this in mind when communicating; it may be appropriate to involve family or carers (with consent). It's probably also worth revising how to perform a mental state assessment and having a working knowledge of the Mental Capacity Act (2007). You may need to advise elderly patients or their carers about community support services such as meals on wheels, the local pharmacist who can deliver a dosette box, home care, domiciliary podiatry or hearing aids. In addition, make sure that you feel comfortable discussing the practicalities of different types of residential and nursing accommodation.

Paediatric patients
Case A7 🎥

Paediatric cases are usually consultations with a parent about a child (though since November 2013 the RCGP will be including a very limited amount of child role players). Usually, though, paediatric cases are achieved through a third party (a parent). If you feel it would be important to examine the child at some point, then explain that you would like to do that and progress with the consultation. You will not gain any marks by spending ages insisting on seeing the child who is not there and not getting on with the consultation.

Teenage contraception, confidentiality and Gillick competency are exam favourites; you would be wise to revise those rules. If you think there has been any illegal activity (for example, under-age sex), then it's important to make it clear (if appropriate) that you're aware of it, whatever you plan to do about it.

[Shaleen: It would be important to establish the age of the partner to identify any potential abuse. You would also need to assess their social support and say that it is illegal to have under-age sex, while maintaining rapport and building trust, which is difficult!]

Finally, it is essential to be alert to the range of presentations of potential child abuse. It can be helpful to adopt a family-centred approach to children, and don't forget that the members of the wider primary healthcare team are available to help manage difficult cases (for example, health visitors, school nurses or child psychologists).

Angry patients
Case B4 🎥

Angry patients can be among the most difficult consultations, both in real life and in the CSA exam.

A good rule of thumb is to apologise for any perceived mistakes or misunderstandings. If you know you have made a mistake, then the advice is to say so early on with a sincere apology. If it's not yet clear if you, or someone else, has made a mistake, then you can still say sorry without apportioning any blame: you can apologise that what has happened has made the patient feel angry. For example, 'I am very sorry that you feel this way.'

If this is said empathetically, it can often defuse a potentially sticky situation, along with adopting a soft tone, maintaining eye contact and never raising your position or voice to match an angry patient's. A calm, open approach from the doctor throughout a difficult consultation will help to settle the patient. Open, relaxed, non-verbal communication and body language are particularly important. Saying 'calm down' to an angry patient nearly always makes matters worse.

A patient may also come in angry about a colleague of yours or a system error in the practice. It is important to listen to the patient's concerns, make sure that they know you are taking them seriously and outline your plan of action. This might include gathering more information, reviewing a doctor or system within a practice, having a significant event meeting or explaining the complaints procedure to the patient in detail. It could also result in additional training for practice staff.

[Shaleen I read my practice complaints procedure patient leaflet and had a mini-tutorial with the practice manager. He went through some of the recent complaints at the practice and how they were dealt with.]

Commonly used techniques in dealing with angry patients are reflection and (often more powerful) legitimisation:

- **Reflection** enables the patient to understand that you have heard their concern and acts as a summary: 'OK, you're angry because you saw the receptionist looking into your medical records.'
- **Legitimisation** is where you recognize the patient's anger by reflecting it back *and* verbally acknowledging its legitimacy: 'So you saw the receptionist looking into your medical records. I can completely understand why you would be upset about that.'

Demanding patients

Patients often make demands of their GP – reasonably or otherwise – and it's the sort of scenario you may well come across in the CSA. A specific demand for something you feel uncomfortable about (for example, an inappropriate prescription or referral) can be tackled effectively by adopting a 'Yes… but no' approach. For example:

Patient: 'Doctor, it's straightforward. I just want to see a dermatologist for my eczema.'
Doctor: 'Yes, of course we can arrange that if it's needed. Now tell me more about your skin.'

If the doctor replied with an immediate 'No', she would effectively remove all hope for the patient and this could escalate to open confrontation. Instead, by using the 'Yes… but' approach the doctor keeps channels of communication open without promising the world. The doctor's response suggests that she would refer the patient if necessary (which is true), but that she needs to move the consultation forward to find out more first.

Another tip for dealing with demands is to 'show the patient your thinking' – just as you might 'show your working' in a maths exam at school. In other words, explain out loud the internal arguments going on in your mind. For example, make it clear that you want to help the patient as much as you can, but also say why you are reluctant to prescribe something inappropriate. This allows the patient to see the problem from your point of view, and your honesty and transparency often go a long way to building trust.

Here's an example where a doctor responds to an inappropriate request for more benzodiazepines for insomnia:

Doctor: 'OK, so can I tell you what I'm thinking? On the one hand I do understand why you've asked for those sleeping tablets again – you're clearly struggling to get enough good-quality sleep, and they've helped you in the short term before. I am very keen to help you get a better night's sleep. On the other hand, the specific pills you've asked for are not recommended for insomnia long term. For example, they can be addictive; they make people feel drowsy the next day, which can affect driving; and they can have withdrawal effects. My dilemma is that by prescribing you this, I would be going against current best practice, which is very clear. We can offer you the same or better improvements with your sleep using different and safer approaches.'

Most reasonable patients are likely to respond to this by engaging with your dilemma – even suggesting reasonable alternatives. Of course, it's not always appropriate to say out loud what you're thinking, but sometimes, if you judge it right, it can encourage a genuinely constructive dialogue rather than a prickly confrontation.

Language barriers

Language barriers can add an extra layer of complexity to a consultation. They do, however, reflect real-life situations, so being sensitive to someone whose first language is not English is important. If interpreters are available then they can be used, as can family members or friends to help translate, but be wary about sensitive questions; signposting becomes particularly important here.

In the exam situation it is more likely that you will come across a patient with good enough English to get through a consultation, but with enough of a language barrier to require particularly clear communication from the doctor. The examiners will be looking for candidates who are non-judgmental and avoid jargon in their explanations. A good tip is to summarise your understanding of what the patient has told you, and then to check their understanding once you have explained a condition or agreed a shared management plan.

Breaking bad news

This situation may come up for some candidates – if it does, you will need to be sensitive. In general, it's often a good idea to start by asking if there's anyone in the waiting area whom the patient would like to be present during the consultation. Check what the patient already knows about the situation so that you are fully up to speed on what's happening and can tailor your message to the patient's level of understanding. While patients often want to be told at the start that you have bad news, don't bombard them with lots of information. Asking them how much they want to know can also tailor your explanation.

These are some common errors in these circumstances:

- Avoiding the issue/putting it off.
- Avoiding cues.
- Avoiding emotional issues.
- Being economical with the truth.
- Being excessively gloomy.
- Being specific with the prognosis (in general, all patients want to know their diagnosis, but only a few want specific questions answered about their prognosis).
- Giving too much information.
- Removing all hope.

Remember that it may be appropriate to say the word 'cancer' if that is a very likely diagnosis; but be aware that after that, patients may not hear anything else. One approach to breaking bad news is summarised by the acronym SPIKES (2). This consists of six steps:

Setting up the interview (allowing enough time; in an appropriate environment; do they wish others to be present?).

Perception (what does the patient know so far: 'Do you know why we have done a scan?').

Invitation (how much does the patient want to know?).

Knowledge (a warning shot that you are about to deliver bad news may be helpful, for example, 'Unfortunately I have some bad news for you…'; delivering the information in small, non-jargon chunks can help).

Emotion (responding to the patient's emotional response).

Strategy and **S**ummary (summarising the information so far, and if appropriate giving them a clear plan of what is going to happen next).

Health promotion

Some CSA cases might present an opportunity for health promotion (think about smoking cessation, obesity, childhood vaccination, smears, alcohol advice and so on). Taking smoking as an illustration, if it seemed relevant within a case predominantly about something else, we would suggest enquiring about the patient's smoking habits and, if appropriate, asking the patient about their readiness to quit or cut down. Depending on their response, you might then offer brief advice and help in how to take the next steps (for example, seeing the smoking-cessation nurse or providing details of the local Alcoholics Anonymous or rehabilitation team). You could also advise the patient that the best way to give up smoking is with an NHS smoking-cessation service.

If the focus of the station is not really about this, then the actor will probably not seem terribly interested and you should not pursue things too far. You can usually trust the actor not to lead you down the garden path – if they are moving you on, then don't waste time dwelling on health promotion, as you're unlikely to score marks and it will eat up your valuable time.

Diversity
Case C5 🎥
As a final point, as GPs we see patients from all walks of life, including those from different cultural backgrounds or sexual identity, for example. The CSA exam tries to reflect this. So be sensitive to any cultural or personal issues that may have a bearing on the consultation. Examiners will be looking for an open-minded, non-judgemental and supportive approach.

References
1. Cupples, M.E., Hart, P.M., Johnston, A. & Jackson, A.J. (2012) Improving healthcare access for people with visual impairment and blindness. *British Medical Journal*, 344, e542.
2. Baile, W.F., Buckman, R., Lenzi, R., Glober, G., Beale, E. & Kudelka, A. (2000) SPIKES – A six-step protocol for delivering bad news: Application to the patient with cancer. *The Oncologist*, 5 (4), 302–311.

Further reading
Breaking Bad News. (A pharma-sponsored website that provides healthcare professionals with suggestions and guidelines on how best to communicate bad news to patients and relatives.) www.breakingbadnews.co.uk.

6 How to Use the CSA Practice Cases

A guide to using the practice cases and the DVD, and a blueprint mapping cases to the RCGP curriculum

You can read the practice cases on your own, but we think it's best to use them in a small group of a minimum of three to four people. One of you should be the doctor, one the patient and another the examiner (Figure 6.1). Having more than one observer is fine. The roles should be rotated after every case or, once the group is functioning well, having one of you play the doctor for a couple of cases in a row may replicate some of the pressure that occurs in the real exam.

We would suggest that you don't look at the cases before you practise them; this makes it more like the real thing for you. We would suggest you have two copies of this book. Whichever of you is playing the patient should have five minutes to read and digest the **patient brief**. Whoever is playing the doctor should only be allowed a couple of minutes to read the short **patient details** and relevant past history – as in the real exam. This would involve you covering up the boxes after details of the patient, otherwise you would know the crux of the case.

Ideally, you should treat the cases like a real exam, with no interaction with the examiner or observer (apart from any examination findings) and no time-outs for help. But to start with, in newly formed groups, it may feel safer to trial cases as a group (one of you plays the patient and the rest of you play the doctor, but taking it in turns when you get stuck).

If there are any notes for the examiner over any particular examination findings, then they are included in the **examination findings** section, but only the parts requested should be handed over to the doctor when they are mentioned. There

How to Pass the CSA Exam, First Edition. Imtiaz Ahmad, Raj Nair, Martin Block and Graham Easton.
© 2015 John Wiley & Sons, Ltd. Published 2015 by John Wiley & Sons, Ltd.

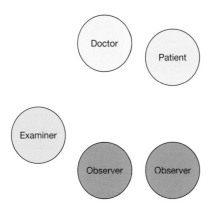

Figure 6.1 Suggested set-up for role playing practice cases as a group.

may not be anything to examine, though, and in this case no other interaction between the doctor and examiner should take place. In the actual exam, any examination findings are sent to the candidate's iPad if requested. It's unlikely you will be able to reproduce this within your small groups, but you could write down the examination findings on a piece of paper or the examiner could just read out any positive examination findings during the consultation. This is what we have done in the DVD.

The examiner or observer should time 10 minutes exactly. As with the real exam, you should not have a warning over how much time is left, but as the doctor you may have a timer in front of you as long as you bring it to the exam!

We would suggest that, to start with at least, you structure your feedback

according to Pendleton's rules (1), given in the tip box as adapted for our practice cases.

However, with time, and a functional group, you could quickly switch to direct comments from the examiner and observers (but always offering constructive suggestions, or highlighting what went well first).

After the details of the case, you will find some brief **key points** about the case that could be a trigger for discussion, and there's also a simple summary grid for **suggested marking criteria** for the examiner to use during the consultation and guide discussion afterwards.

The more detailed information on each case (**trainer's feedback**) is worth reading individually at the end of the session to help consolidate the information that you've processed that day. We would suggest not doing more than four cases in a row without a break, or a chance to debrief in detail, either individually or as a group.

Please bear in mind that our guidance and comments on the suggested marking criteria reflect our opinions as experienced GP educators; this is not an RCGP marking scheme, and cannot of course guarantee to match what the RCGP examiners' criteria might be for each particular case. But our comments are based on our years of experience with trainees preparing and passing the exam. As in real-life general practice, different GPs may have different views on the same case – you may disagree with us on some cases, which is fine. The real value lies in you discussing and debating with your colleagues what you would count as pass/fail.

The cases we have written have all been tried and tested by previous trainees on our CSA preparation courses, and adjusted where necessary in response to their feedback. We hope that means they'll work without a hitch – but please let us know if you think of any improvements we could incorporate for the next edition.

Using the DVD practice cases

The 12 cases on the DVD are all taken from cases in Chapter 7 in this book, where they are highlighted with this symbol:

We hope that they will provide useful raw material for you to watch alone, or to discuss as a group. Each consultation is accompanied by a five-minute feedback discussion between the trainer (one of the authors) and the 'trainee' (one of our

recent GP ST3s). And if you want some really useful tips from doctors who have recently sat the exam, watch the half-hour round-table discussion.

Our friendly GP ST3s had not seen the cases before we filmed them, 'as live', in the surgery with simulated actor patients who had been given the actor briefs beforehand. As far as possible we created CSA conditions for them – a minute or two to read their brief, strictly 10 minutes' duration for the consultation (with a buzzer sounding to end it) and any examination results handed to them by the examiner (we used paper rather than iPads).

During each consultation, we have added brief comments as 'subtitles', some of which might be about consultation skills in general, but most of which are examples of specific indicators for each of the three CSA assessment domains. We have adopted the same colour coding as the RCGP uses in its document *Generic Indicators for Targeted Assessment Domains*:

• Data gathering, technical and assessment skills
• Clinical management skills
• Interpersonal skills

We haven't commented on every single example, but we have tried to highlight the ones that stood out for us.

You can use the DVD cases in whichever way you find most helpful. But we suspect the real value will be in reflecting on what worked well and what could have been done better, then seeing how your thoughts compare to ours in the feedback discussion afterwards. The feedback discussions followed immediately after the consultations and, of course, they are our own views – they don't claim to reflect exactly how an examiner would mark the consultation. Nevertheless, as already stated, they do reflect our years of collective experience running preparation courses for the CSA and preparing our ST3s for success in the exam.

You could watch the DVDs alone, or as a group. You could also then read our detailed feedback notes for each case in the book, including following up further reading or references if needed.

Developing your own cases

A great way to learn more is to write your own CSA cases to practise in your groups. We would advise you to use the blank case template as a pro-forma (see Appendix 6.1).

When writing a case decide:

• Which part of the GP curriculum this case relates to (see Appendix 6.2)

• Why is the patient consulting now? What are their ideas, concerns and expectations?

• What is the particular challenge of this case?

• What is the patient's story?

• What are the examination findings?

• What would constitute a pass or fail in each of the domains (data gathering, clinical management and interpersonal skills)? Remember, good cases should reflect real-life general practice. Use our cases as a guide, and enjoy writing your own.

Reference

1. Pendleton, D., Schofield, T., Tate, P. & Havelock, P. (2003) *The Consultation: An Approach to Learning and Teaching.* Oxford: Oxford University Press.

Further reading

Cantillon, P. & Sargeant, J. (2008) Giving feedback in clinical settings. *British Medical Journal*, 337, 1292–1294.

Appendix 6.1: Template for writing your own practice cases

CASE: ....(e.g. Itchy Bottom)

PATIENT

Name:

Age:

PMH:

DH:

Other information for doctor (e.g. recent consultations):

Patient brief:

Opening remarks: '..........'

Patient's agenda:

EXAMINATION FINDINGS

REFLECTION

Key points:

Data gathering:

Management:

Interpersonal skills:

Suggested marking criteria:

	Clear Pass	Pass	Fail	Clear Fail
Data gathering				
Management				
Interpersonal skills				

Appendix 6.2: Curriculum coverage

Clinical Skills Assessment Case Selection Blueprint	Primary nature of case					
Primary system or area of disease →	Acute Illness	Chronic Illness	Undifferentiated Illness	Psycho- social	Preventive/ lifestyle	Other
Genetics				Paternity test (B9)		
Paediatrics		Sickle cell (C10) Nocturnal enuresis (B11)		CP (A3)		
Elderly medicine	Hearing loss (B5)			Elder abuse (C2)		
Women's health	PE post C-section (B·2)		PCOS (A2)	FGM (C5)	Antenatal booking (A1)	
Men's health				ED (B6)	PSA testing (C4)	
Sexual health	STI (B3)	HIV (C8)				
End-of-life care				Palliative care (A12)		
Mental heath problems	Acute stress (A13)		Gambling (C3)	Insomnia (B8)		
Learning difficulties	Breast lump C6)					
Cardiovascular	Chest pain (A3)	HTN (A5)				
Gastrointestinal			IBS (B1)			

(Continued)

Appendix 6.2: (Continued)

Clinical Skills Assessment Case Selection Blueprint	Primary nature of case					
Primary system or area of disease ↓	Acute Illness	Chronic Illness	Undifferentiated Illness	Psycho- social	Preventive/ lifestyle	Other
Misuse of drugs and alcohol				Drug withdrawal (A8)		
ENT	URTI (A11)	Allergic Rhinitis (B13)				
Ophthalmology	Acute red eye (C13)					
Metabolic	Acute DM2 (C11)	DM2 (A6)				
Neurological		MS (B10)		Headache (C1)		
Respiratory	COPD exacerbation (C7) PE post-C section (B12)	Asthma (C12)				
Musculoskeletal	Gout (A4)			Back pain (B2)	Obesity in knee pain (B7)	
Dermatology		Paediatric eczema (A9)				
Urological			Renal colic (A10)	Nocturnal Enuresis (B11)		
Oncology	Palliative care (A12)					
Other					Inappropriate sick note	Confidentiality (B4)

7 CSA Practice Cases

Cases (A)

1 Antenatal booking appointment
2 Polycystic Ovarian Syndrome (PCOS) 📹
3 Chest pain (musculoskeletal) 📹
4 Gout 📹
5 New onset hypertension
6 Type 2 diabetes
7 Child protection
8 Drug withdrawal
9 Paediatric eczema
10 Renal colic 📹
11 Upper respiratory tract infection 📹
12 Palliative care 📹
13 Acute stress 📹

All patient names and details in the practice cases are fictional - any resemblance to any real patient, living or dead, is purely coincidental.

How to Pass the CSA Exam, First Edition. Imtiaz Ahmad, Raj Nair, Martin Block and Graham Easton.
© 2015 John Wiley & Sons, Ltd. Published 2015 by John Wiley & Sons, Ltd.

Case A1

PATIENT
Name: Mrs Anne Cole
Age: 33
SH: Never smoked, drinks alcohol occasionally but not planning on drinking any more
PMH: Hayfever, fracture of radius 5 years ago
DH: Microgynon OCP (stopped 1 year ago); folic acid 400 mcg

A1 Antenatal booking appointment

Patient brief: Mrs Anne Cole

You have just discovered you are pregnant and have come to the GP to book your pregnancy care. You have been trying for a baby for around 8 months, you are in a happy marriage and you are excited about the pregnancy. Your last period was 6 weeks ago and you have done a pregnancy test, which was positive.

You have been pregnant only once before, in your 20s, when you were in a new relationship. You had the pregnancy terminated surgically and, if asked, you are slightly concerned whether that could affect this pregnancy. If asked, you have had chicken pox as a child but are not sure about rubella. Your partner is supportive. You think it's worth increasing the amount you're eating because you're now 'eating for two'.

Patient's opening remarks: *'I've just found out I'm pregnant…'*

Patient's agenda: You have come to book your pregnancy. If asked, you are interested in knowing what things you should avoid in your diet. You are aware that being pregnant will have an effect on your life, but you are happy about that.

EXAMINATION FINDINGS

BMI 26
BP 112/78
Urine dipstick NAD
Pregnancy test positive if asked

Reflection

Key points

- **Data gathering:** Taking a previous obstetric history and dating the pregnancy are important, and you should calculate BMI and BP as a minimum.
- **Management:** Key information to be discussed with the patient (once she has had a chance to share what she knows already) would include diet, smoking, alcohol, vitamin supplementation, scans and midwife appointments.
- **Interpersonal skills:** Responding appropriately and in a non-judgemental style to the patient's opening statement of 'Doctor, I think I'm pregnant' is important both to form rapport and also to find out her intentions with the pregnancy. Exploring the patient's social history with particular attention to any relationships she may have is also key.

Suggested marking criteria

	Clear Pass	Pass	Fail	Clear Fail
Data gathering	Social history established	PMH, obstetric history and current mood established; takes BMI	No social history established, dating the pregnancy correctly, no BMI measured	No previous obstetric or past medical history gathered
Management	Explains clearly what will happen during antenatal care and scans	Gives majority of advice	No advice re alcohol or scans	No advice re diet, smoking or vitamin supplementation
Interpersonal skills	Delivers information in bite-size chunks and summarises at the end	Picks up cues	Fails to pick up cues, e.g. worries over past termination of pregnancy, concerns over diet	Didactic style of consulting with no emotion showing towards patient

Trainer's comments

Don't make assumptions. When the patient announces she is pregnant, despite her looking happy, it is important for the doctor not to assume what her intentions are with the pregnancy. If the doctor were to react with a statement of 'congratulations', this may not go down well with a patient who intended to terminate the pregnancy. However, once the doctor has established this is something the patient is happy about, it is entirely appropriate to convey your good wishes to the patient. Once the opening exchanges are over, you need to establish some facts in order to perform well on the station.

It's important to estimate last menstrual period (LMP) **to date the pregnancy** and give an estimated date of confinement.

Enquiring about any **previous pregnancies** needs to be handled quite delicately, especially when the patient reveals she had a previous termination. It is important for the doctor not to be judgemental but also to be clear about the previous termination not affecting the current pregnancy. Reacting to the non-verbal cues the patient gives about her fears over the previous termination of pregnancy would distinguish between a good and excellent candidate.

Social history is important: Does she have a partner? Is he or she supportive? Are there any problems in the relationship? If there is a hint that there are, then further questioning along with direct questions regarding domestic violence are recommended. You could start with an open question of 'How are things with your partner?'. The next stage of enquiry is often difficult to phrase and much relies on softer skills like listening, eye contact and tone, but something along the lines of 'Has your partner ever abused you?' or 'Do you live in fear of your partner?' could be approaches to try.

Enquiring about her **mood** is also important. This can be done simply by observing the patient, but for the purposes of the exam, by directly asking how she feels about being pregnant. If at all worried, delving deeper is appropriate and you could use the standard (NICE) depression screening questions (1):

- During the last month, have you been feeling down, depressed or hopeless?
- During the last month, have you often been bothered by having little pleasure or interest in doing things?

Even if not prompted, the doctor should volunteer **lifestyle information** to the patient once they have established what the patient knows:

- **Diet:** A reasonable selection of the following could be discussed: avoid unpasteurised cheeses (risk of listeria); no more than two portions of oily fish a week (risk of mercury building up, which could affect the growing foetus); avoid raw shellfish; eggs must be cooked thoroughly (so avoid home-made mayonnaise/mousse); avoid animal liver or liver pâté (build-up of potentially toxic vitamin A); ensure meat is thoroughly cooked; wash vegetables and fruit thoroughly. You could direct the patient to the Department of Health website (2) for further precise information.
- **Smoking status:** If the patient does smoke, offer appropriate cessation advice with onward referral to a cessation adviser who specialises in pregnancy; note that nicotine replacement therapy is permitted to be used in pregnancy as long as the risks and benefits are explained to the patient. No other drug (buproprion or varenicline) is currently licensed or recommended for use in pregnancy. The NICE guidance (3) has more details.

- **Alcohol:** If consumed, should be minimal and no binges.
- **Exercise:** Good for health and relaxation. Walking, swimming and yoga are OK. Avoid strenuous exercise or contact sports.

Given the patient's high **BMI**, it may be helpful to discuss with her the recommended calorie intake at her stage of pregnancy (women are not 'eating for two' until the last trimester, when they are recommended to consume only 200 extra calories a day). If clinically obese (BMI > 30), patients should not try to lose weight but eat healthily and exercise regularly with a view to avoid gaining weight. Remember, obese women are at a higher risk of complications and should be started on high-dose folic acid (5 mg daily), which would need to be prescribed (in addition to their over-the-counter low-dose folic acid/vitamin D). Some obstetricians start such patients on low-dose aspirin from the first trimester.

There is a week 11–14 nuchal dating **scan** that, along with the quadruple blood test, can give an estimate of Down's syndrome risk, which may or may not be important to the woman. It is unlikely that you would be probed much on this in this station as there is a lot to be covered, but in another station you may need to know about further steps (amniocentesis and CVS) that could be offered to women at high risk. There is an additional anomaly scan at 18–20 weeks of pregnancy.

Following the Chief Medical Officer's (CMO) letter from the Department of Health in 2012 (4), women are now advised to take a **vitamin supplement** that contains both vitamin D and folic acid; this could be prescribed or purchased or supplied from Sure Start (if operating in the area).

Explain that you will fill in a form (**FW8**) so that the patient can claim free NHS prescriptions (should she need them); NHS dental and eye services should also be mentioned. As with prescriptions, it is probably best not actually to fill in the form, but to make it clear to the examiner that you are doing so.

Summarising the key features of this busy consultation (in particular highlighting when to expect the scans and appointments to come through) would be important here.

It is useful to give the patient an idea of when to expect scans and **follow-up antenatal appointments** (ten for uncomplicated nulliparous women, seven for multiparous).

References

1. National Institute for Health and Clinical Excellence (2009) *Depression in Adults*. London: NICE. http://guidance.nice.org.uk/CG90
2. Department of Health information on diet in pregnancy. http://www.nhs.uk/chq/Pages/917.aspx?CategoryID=54&SubCategoryID=130#close
3. National Institute for Health and Clinical Excellence (2010) *How to Stop Smoking in Pregnancy and Childbirth*. London: NICE. http://www.

nice.org.uk/nicemedia/live/13023/
49346/49346.pdf

4. Chief Medical Officer letter on vitamin D supplementation in pregnancy, babies and the elderly (2012). http://www.dh. gov.uk/prod_consum_dh/groups/dh_ digitalassets/@dh/@en/documents/ digitalasset/dh_132508.pdf

Further Reading

National Institute for Health and Clinical Excellence (2008) *Antenatal Care – Routine Care for the Healthy Pregnant Woman*. London: NICE. http://www.nice. org.uk/nicemedia/live/11947/40110/ 40110.pdf

---

PATIENT

Name: Ms Pauline Smithye
Age: 24
PMH: Acne
DH: Clindamycin/benzoyl peroxide cream

A2 Polycystic Ovarian Syndrome (PCOS)

Patient brief: Ms Pauline Smithye

You are a 24-year-old trainee lawyer. You have always had problems with your periods, which started when you were aged 13. They have always been irregular and you thought this was normal, until you moved in with a few female work colleagues and realised that they all have regular periods and that yours are not right.

Your periods are generally quite light and difficult to predict. Sometimes they come every 2 or 3 months. You have no bleeding between periods and you are currently not sexually active but have had sex before (if asked, the last occasion was a few months ago). You have never had any risky contacts and have always used condoms; your last partner was 3 months ago. You have never had a smear test. Your last menstrual period was about 6 weeks ago.

You take an effective cream for acne but have no other medical problems. If asked, you do get a bit more hair on your face than your peers. Though embarrassing, you don't need any treatment for this as you have an excellent beautician who works wonders for you.

You have never been pregnant and have never had any tests for sexual transmitted infections, but would be happy to do these if asked. If asked, you are worried about your fertility, as your mother went through the menopause in her early 30s and you have always wanted to have a child. You are worried about leaving starting a family late, but you don't have a partner currently and are not financially secure, in contrast to most of your peers, so this is not an option. You have no menopausal symptoms.

There is no other family medical history. All is fine at work otherwise.

Patient's opening remarks: *'Yes, my periods are a bit weird at the moment, so I thought I'd better come and see you.'*

Patient's agenda: You would like to know what potential problems you could have and what the doctor could do to help.

Reflection

Key points

- **Data gathering:** There is a lot to do in this station, but ruling out red flag symptoms (IMB/PCB) as well as performing a pregnancy test are essential to pass. Allowing the actress to help guide you towards the psychosocial elements of the consultation should allow you to focus less on the physical problems and more on the patient's worries. Having said that, eliciting a history of hirsutism and acne, along with the irregularity of her periods, would help point towards PCOS.

- **Management:** Performing a pelvic exam is not essential here, but mentioning follow-up for this and or any appropriate investigations (transvaginal ultrasound [TV USS], bloods) would be important.

Suggested marking criteria

	Clear Pass	Pass	Fail	Clear Fail
Data gathering	Establishes pattern of periods, acne and hirsutism	Sends off STI screen	Does not perform a pregnancy test	Does not take a history of intermenstrual/ postcoital bleeding
Management	Deals with fears of fertility, arranging appropriate follow-up	Explains potential diagnoses	Only arranges bloods +/- TV USS with no further explanation of potential diagnosis	No tests arranged
Interpersonal skills	Delivers information in bite-size chunks and summarises at the end	Picks up on cues	Fails to pick up cues, e.g. worries over fertility	Didactic style of consulting with no emotion shown towards the patient

Trainer's comments

There is a lot to do in this station. The gynaecology history here does not need to be exhaustive, but ought to **establish the pattern of the patient's periods**. Ensuring there are no **red flag symptoms** (of intermenstrual/postcoital bleeding) is important. Irregular periods in a woman who has been or is sexually active (with no adequate contraception) ought to prompt you to ask for a **pregnancy test** to rule out an ectopic pregnancy. Likewise, considering screening for **sexually transmitted infections** (STI) would be prudent given the patient's demographics.

The history of acne ought to prompt you to measure the patient's BMI to **consider PCOS**. It would be worth asking about hirsutism.

A major conundrum here is **what can be achieved in today's appointment** and what can be postponed for the follow-up. One approach could be to rule out pregnancy, send some self-screening swabs for an STI screen and bring the patient back to do a formal pelvic exam and arrange blood tests (for example, luteinising hormone [LH], follicle-stimulating hormone [FSH], sex hormone-binding globulin [SHBG], oestradiol and testosterone) with or without a pelvic scan. Some candidates may choose to do all of this in one consultation, but this may be unrealistic in 10 minutes. A diagnosis of PCOS can be made on the basis of two out of three criteria (cysts on scan; bloods indicative of PCOS; symptoms of PCOS), so doing all these investigations on the first visit may at the least be a waste of resources; however, more importantly for the exam, it may use up valuable time that you could use to explore the patient's fears (of infertility) and form rapport.

This station will differentiate the good from the excellent, and the novice from the experienced consulter. Although in hospital you might be encouraged to cover all the investigations in one visit, in general practice sometimes less is more. Here, postponing some elements of the consultation allows you to focus on the more psychosocial aspects, but it takes skill and guts. It isn't always the best approach, though, so how do you know when to focus more on the psychosocial aspects or the biomedical aspects of a consultation?

Our advice would be to enquire about some of the psychosocial aspects of the consultation early on and be guided by the role player. If there isn't much mileage in this line of enquiry, the actor patient is likely to give you cues to make that clear. For example, they may say something like '*No, that's all completely fine. I just want to know what the problem is*.' Once your history has ruled out the key red flags and you have ruled out an ectopic pregnancy with a pregnancy test, how the consultation plays out will be dependent on the candidate. Focusing on the psychosocial will probably lead to more marks – the other investigations could be mentioned, with full discussion postponed until next time.

Don't forget that if you want to perform a pelvic exam, you should **offer a chaperone**. As the patient wants to know potential diagnoses, you could explain that you wish to rule out STI with a self-screening swab or urine test today, and that the other possibility could be PCOS, so you would like to bring the patient back to examine her or do bloods and a scan.

You can practise explaining PCOS guided by patient information leaflets such as those from www.patient.co.uk (1).

Reference

1. Patient UK information leaflets. www.patient.co.uk

Further Reading

NICE Clinical Knowledge Summary, PCOS, updated February 2013. http://cks.nice.org.uk/polycystic-ovary-syndrome#!topicsummary

Case A3 📷

A3 Chest pain (musculoskeletal)

Patient brief: Mr Josh Sanders

You are a stressed 33-year-old single lawyer who works long hours in the city. You are coping, but lately you have been experiencing sharp left-sided chest pain, which is worse when you are moving or taking deep breaths.

If asked, you go to the gym five times a week and find the treadmill helpful in dealing with the stress (which you do not need further help with). You do not experience any chest pain when exercising. There are no associated symptoms that go along with this (no shortness of breath, nausea, coughing up blood or sweating, for example).

The pain can last hours and you have had it most days in the last month. You have not taken anything to help.

No one else in the family has heart disease. You drink and smoke socially only. You are not keen to give up either. You do not feel down or depressed and you sleep well.

Patient's opening remarks: '*I'm a bit worried about this chest pain I've been getting, doctor.*'

Patient's agenda: If asked, you are worried it could be your heart, as your father died of a heart attack aged 62.

+---+
| **EXAMINATION FINDINGS** |
| If asked: |
| Heart sounds normal |
| HR 78 reg |
| BP 112/78 |
| Slight left lower rib tenderness |
| Chest clear |
| Oxygen saturations 98% on room air |
+---+

Reflection

Key points

- **Data gathering:** Important to rule out any serious cardiac or respiratory conditions.
- **Management:** Exploring the patient's fears of ischaemic heart disease (IHD) and managing these would again distinguish between a pass and fail here.

- **Interpersonal skills:** Having asked a few open questions, use several key closed questions to cover red flags and help formulate a differential diagnosis. Exploring the patient's psychosocial history and delving into any lifestyle advice would be good practice, but trust the actor not to lead you too far if this is not relevant.

Suggested marking criteria

	Clear Pass	Pass	Fail	Clear Fail
Data gathering	Takes oxygen saturations, elicits fears of IHD	Establishes the pain is not present on exercising and stress at work	Does not ask about risk factors for heart disease	Does not examine the patient
Management	Offers smoking-cessation advice and help with stress	Offers NSAIDs (but checks no contraindications) and puts the patient's fears of IHD at rest	Does not explain the likely diagnosis or put the patient's fears of IHD at rest	Does not order any investigations
Interpersonal skills	Delivers information in bite-size chunks and summarises at the end	Picks up cues	Fails to pick up cues, for example, worries over IHD	Didactic style of consulting with no emotion shown towards the patient

Trainer's comments

Clearly, in a chest pain station it is important to ask several key questions. Having started the station with some open questions, ask some specific questions to direct your differential diagnosis and **rule out red flags**. To make this flow better, you could **signpost** with something like: 'I would like to ask

you several specific questions, if that's OK?' Then ask questions such as the following:

- What does the pain feel like? Where is it? What brings it on and relieves it?
- Do you have any symptoms at the same time (shortness of breath, nausea, vomiting, sweating, coughing up blood or feel very unwell with it)?

- Do you smoke? If the patient does smoke, explore their readiness to quit and offer cessation advice if the patient wants it (but do not push this if it is declined). The actor will lead you here.
- Is there any history of heart problems or strokes in your family? (For example, significant history includes first-degree relative under the age of 60 having a cardiac event or stroke.)
- Enquire about risk factors for pulmonary embolism (PE; for example, clotting disorders, recent fight or personal or family history).

The fact that the pain is not present when the patient exercises should make an ischaemic cause very unlikely, but for the interpersonal skills domain it is also important to find out **what the patient believes** the pain may be due to or is concerned about. Eliciting and managing the fear that it might be a heart attack would distinguish between a pass and a fail in the clinical management domain.

Examining for heart sounds, blood pressure, heart rate and feeling for local chest wall tenderness is important, but remember that tenderness may also be present in a PE. Addressing the patient's fears and giving clear advice about treatment plans like non-steroidal anti-inflammatories (NSAIDs; checking there is no common contraindication such as asthma, chronic kidney disease, gastric ulcer) would also be important. Exploring the patient's **psychosocial history**, paying particular attention to his occupation and ways of coping with any perceived stress, would distinguish a pass from a fail in data gathering. Offering any help with this would be good practice, but trust the actor not to lead you too far down this path if there are no marks there (as in this case).

Case A4 📖

> ### PATIENT
>
> **Name:** Mr Paul Smith
> **Age:** 42
> **SH:** Never smoked, drinks 20 units alcohol/week
> **PMH:** Hypertension; appendectomy 1992
> **DH:** Indapamide 1.5 mg; no allergies

A4 Gout

> **Patient brief: Mr Paul Smith**
>
> You are a 42-year-old labourer and you have had a swollen thumb for the past 48 hours. It has been red and hot. It hurts to move it, but you are able to do this. You have had this a couple of times before in the same area, but this time it has lasted a little longer and hurts more. You feel well and have not had a fever. Your other joints do not cause you problems and your mother has some form of arthritis, which only started a few years ago; she only takes painkillers for it and her doctor says it's old age.
>
> Work is fine and you do enjoy a few pints of beer with your colleagues after work. You are aware that your diet is not great and have been considering altering it, especially if it would prevent this joint problem.
>
> You are separated from your ex-wife, with whom you have a 5-year-old son. You live alone and are currently single. You do not feel capable of working and wonder how to certify your sick leave, as you have never done this before. You have taken the last 2 days off work and will return once your symptoms improve. There is no other work your manager could give you that does not involve manual labour and you are in too much pain to do this. You have not had any weakness, numbness or stiffness of any joints and your symptoms occur equally throughout the day. Your weight has been stable.
>
> **Patient's opening remarks:** '*It's about my thumb, doctor. It's causing me a few problems. I can't even go to work. So I thought should come and see what's going on, you know…*'
>
> **Patient's agenda:** You want to know what this is, how you can prevent it happening again and long term whether there is anything that could stop it altogether.

EXAMINATION FINDINGS

If asked:

BP 148/84

Temperature 37 °C

BMI 24

The candidate should be allowed to examine the patient. This should entail inspection and an attempt at active and passive movement of the joint. The actor should be able to move the joint, but it will be painful. A photo of gout will be shown after the examination.

Reflection

Key points

- **Data gathering:** The diagnosis of gout should be relatively straightforward here, but red flag questions and examination to rule out infective and inflammatory causes are important.
- **Management:** You should deal with both the current attack as well as lifestyle advice and the switching of the diuretic medication to an ACE inhibitor. Safety-netting over red flag symptoms is needed to score a pass on communication.
- **Interpersonal skills:** Exploring the effect of the problem on the patient as well as eliciting and dealing with the patient's concerns over future attacks and the need for self-certification would differentiate between a clear pass and a pass for the candidate on data gathering.

Suggested marking criteria

	Clear Pass	Pass	Fail	Clear Fail
Data gathering	Establishes frequency of attacks and patient's concerns	Asks about lifestyle factors that could trigger gout	Inflammatory or infective symptoms or signs	Does not examine the patient
Management	Discusses potential for allopurinol in the future if needed; deals with sick note query	Stops diuretic and gives lifestyle advice; explains the diagnosis clearly	Offers NSAIDs, orders bloods	No treatment or explanation given
Interpersonal skills	Delivers information in bite-size chunks and summarises at the end	Picks up cues, safety-netting	Fails to pick up cues	Does not pick up failing verbal and/or non-verbal cues from the patient

Trainer's comments

Gout is a common primary care condition, and candidates should be familiar with its presentation and management as well as potential differential diagnoses. Ensuring that the joint is not septic (by enquiring about and taking a temperature, and because the joint has some movement) and that there are no inflammatory features (family history, stiffness, early morning symptoms and other joints being fine) is key to **excluding red flags**.

Enquiring about the **effect on the patient**, as well as what they think may have caused the problem and what might help, will differentiate good from excellent candidates.

This is a good opportunity to demonstrate your skills in **explaining a complex condition** clearly to the patient. For example (1): 'Gout causes attacks of painful inflammation (redness, pain, and swelling) in one or more joints. It is a type of arthritis which can be severe. It is caused by a chemical in the blood called uric acid; when the levels of uric acid get too high you can get tiny crystals forming within the joint which cause an attack of gout.'

Handing over information about **dietary triggers** is important (in particular alcohol and red meat). A patient information leaflet would be helpful. The diagnosis here is mainly a clinical one, but some candidates may choose to perform some **baseline blood tests** (for example, full blood count [FBC], urea and electrolytes [U&E], bone profile, diabetes screen and uric acid). Given that this is a repeat episode, this would be warranted.

Ensuring clear arrangements for **follow-up and safety-netting** (to seek medical help if the patient cannot move the joint, other joints are affected or if they develop a temperature) should form part of the management for a candidate to pass. A good candidate would establish that the patient would like to know if there is anything that can be used to stop these attacks. The frequency of attacks would not yet warrant the use of a prophylactic agent (allopurinol), but mentioning that there is a drug that could prevent it from occurring very frequently would be a good idea. **Lifestyle advice** is key in the management here, specifically around diet (reduction in protein and food high in purines and yeast extract such as red meat, seafood and marmite, respectively), as well as cutting down on alcohol.

It is also important to **replace the diuretic** (which can trigger gout) with something like an ACE inhibitor (ACEi), which doesn't precipitate gout and would also be more appropriate for hypertension treatment in a 42-year-old. For all patients, remember to arrange blood tests (U&E) 1–2 weeks after initiating and increasing ACEi doses. Some doctors may choose to use an angiotensin II blocker instead as it is meant to have uricosuric properties, so this might be another alternative.

For the acute pain, as long as there are no contraindications to **NSAIDs**, these should be used. You may choose to hold off starting the ACEi until the patient has finished their NSAID, in order to avoid nephrotoxicity and also to establish baseline renal function. Alternatively, you could use **colchicine**, but you must remember to warn the patient to stop this if they develop toxicity symptoms (for example, gastrointestinal symptoms, especially diarrhoea). The patient's question about what to do for work needs to be tackled and here you could use either a **short-term sick note** (after a 7-day period of self-certification) or a 'fit note' advising amended duties; though this may not be feasible given his work.

Reference

1. Patient UK. Patient information leaflet on gout. http://www.patient.co.uk/health/gout-leaflet

Case A5

PATIENT

Name: Mr Michael Brady
Age: 58
PMH: Nil of note
DH: No regular medication

Consultation notes for two latest consultations by practice nurse:
Ears syringed. BP 159/92. Repeat with me next week.
Repeat BP a week later 158/88, to follow up with GP next week.

A5 New onset hypertension

Patient brief: Mr Michael Brady

You are a 58-year-old retired dock worker who came to the GP surgery last month to get your ear syringed by the practice nurse. Incidentally, she found that your blood pressure was elevated. She advised you to come back a week later to repeat it. Your blood pressure was high again and she advised you to see a GP.

This was a surprise to you, as you had been quite fit when younger, but lately you have not been focused on your health. Your granddaughter has been ill in hospital with leukaemia and you have been spending most of your time helping the family and have needed to drive for a few hours every day to visit her in hospital, as well as helping your son with shopping and household chores. Your wife passed away from breast cancer 3 years ago. You are coping fine, but things are too busy at the moment for you to lead a healthy lifestyle. Things will calm down in a few months, as your granddaughter will be having a bone marrow transplant soon.

You are not depressed and are aware that high blood pressure can cause heart attacks. You would be interested in knowing how you could reduce this through your diet and any other practical advice the doctor can give, but you aren't keen on any significant changes for the next couple of months. In fact, it has been very difficult for you to attend the surgery.

You are otherwise well with no significant past medical problems. Your only relative with heart disease is your father, who had a heart attack aged 58. You drink a glass of wine at weekends with meals. You currently smoke five cigarettes a day, do no exercise and eat takeaways or microwave meals most of the time.

Patient's opening remarks: '*The nurse asked me to come and see you – I think it was about my blood pressure…*'

Patient's agenda: You aren't interested in giving up smoking at the moment with all that is going on, but you would speak to a smoking-cessation adviser once things calm down in your personal life. It is the same situation with exercise, but you could eat more healthily and this could be something simple you could change, if you knew what healthy choices there are.

EXAMINATION FINDINGS

If asked:
BP 158/96
Urine dipstick: NAD
BMI 27.5
Normal fundoscopy

Reflection
Key points

- **Management:** Suggest some simple next investigations (ambulatory or home blood pressure monitoring) and give some practical lifestyle preventative advice (mainly dietary) in bite-size chunks. An empathetic approach to the patient's social situation is paramount. Given the grandchild's pressing illness, it would not be realistic to insist on major changes to this patient's lifestyle right now.

Regarding lifestyle advice, mentioning the need to eat a more Mediterranean diet containing less salt is important. Brief smoking-cessation advice that respects the patient's autonomy is also important. Once it is established that the patient is not keen to give up at the moment, simply signposting to a smoking-cessation adviser would be enough.

In terms of safety-netting, ensuring that the patient understands the importance of booking a follow-up appointment in 2 months is vital. If there is time, check the patient's understanding of the plan; there is a lot of information here.

- **Interpersonal skills:** The key thing in this consultation is to form rapport so the patient will come back once things in their personal life are less hectic. It is important to explain clearly, in terms the patient can relate to, what high blood pressure is and what risks it poses. Picking up on the cues of what is going on with this patient's family is also key. Enquiring what the patient already knows about high blood pressure comes before any explanation that should take into account his background and baseline knowledge. Patient information leaflets can be useful here.

Suggested marking criteria

	Clear Pass	Pass	Fail	
Data gathering	Risk factors for heart disease	Social circumstances; establishes the patient is too busy to undergo full investigations currently	Performs a BMI and takes a family history	
Management	Arranges home BP monitoring and mentions the need later for bloods/ECG	Ensures follow-up and gives practical lifestyle advice on diet in detail; mentions the need to give up smoking	Informs the patient of the need to exercise more	
Interpersonal skills	Summarises at the end; ensures the patient is involved in management plan, i.e. what he can realistically achieve in the short term	Delivers information in bite-size chunks; picks up cues and explains importance of follow-up	Fails to pick up cues, e.g. worries over being able to make significant changes to lifestyle at the moment	

Trainer's comments

Picking up on the cues of what is going on with this patient's family is key, both in terms of gauging the stress he is feeling and what is realistically achievable in this consultation. Given the grand-child's illness, it wouldn't be realistic to insist on major changes to this patient's lifestyle now. There may be further opportunities in a few months.

The key thing in this consultation is to form **rapport** so that the patient will come back once things in his personal life have settled down a bit. In addition, it's important to suggest some basic **investigations**, offer some **lifestyle advice** and explain what high blood pressure is and what the risks are.

Arranging 24-hour ambulatory blood pressure monitoring (ABPM) would be in accordance with NICE guidance (1), but may not be practical for this patient. Taking the blood pressure today and perhaps a urine dipstick test would probably be enough. **Arranging an ECG** would again be good practice, but also unrealistic given current pressures on his time. In addition, not all practices have in-house ECG facilities and arranging a visit to the hospital for this might be even harder for him.

For a clear pass on management, arranging for the patient to take **home blood pressure readings,** which could be brought back in two months once his grandchild has had her transplant, would be as good as ambulatory blood pressure monitoring. This could be done before the next consultation and would not have an impact on the patient's time constraints. You could arrange **fasting blood tests** (for lipid profile, estimated glomerular filtration rate [eGFR] and glucose [or HbA1c]) but that might be equally impractical given the patient's current predicament. Perhaps mentioning that they would need to be done, along with an ECG when time is less pressing for the patient, is enough and shows sensitivity for the patient's personal schedule.

You should try to find out what the patient already knows about high blood pressure before offering a **tailor-made explanation**. One possible general explanation could be: 'Your blood pressure is a measure of the force your heart has to generate to pump blood around the body. If it is too high it can, over time, cause heart attacks and strokes. Having said that, it is one risk factor out of many, including things like cholesterol, smoking, family history, weight and so on.' Many candidates find **patient information leaflets** useful when practising their explanations and for suggesting to patients to take away from the consultation.

It is important to mention the need to eat a more **Mediterranean diet** containing less salt and saturated fat (high in fruit, vegetables, legumes and cereals, fish and white meat instead of red meat; mono-unsaturated oils in place of saturated animal fats; moderate red wine intake with meals). This is the main lifestyle intervention that is practical for the patient, so detail on this would be important. You should note the patient's **smoking status** and offer brief advice that giving up is also paramount to protect the heart. But once you have established that the patient is not keen to give up yet, simply signposting to a smoking cessation adviser would be enough. You would naturally pick this up again at a follow-up appointment.

Ensuring that the patient understands the importance of booking a **follow-up** appointment in two months is vital. If there is time, check that the patient has a **clear understanding** of the follow-up plans; you will have given them a lot of information in this consultation.

Reference

1. National Institute for Health and Clinical Excellence (2011) *Hypertension: Clinical Management of Primary Hypertension in Adults*. London: NICE. http://guidance.nice.org.uk/CG127

Case A6

PATIENT

Name: Mr Steven James

Age: 54

PMH: Type 2 diabetes diagnosed 5 years ago; appendectomy 25 years ago; ex-moderate smoker, gave up 5 years ago

DH: Metformin 500 mg bd, aspirin 75 mg

Last consultation 2 weeks ago (entry by diabetic nurse):

DECS scan arranged, normal foot neurology and pulses. Depression screening questions negative. All is well. Diet/lifestyle discussed. Has been making efforts to lose weight; healthy diet. Flu vaccine advised. BMI 26 (down from 26.1). BP 128/74.

Bloods and review with Dr.

Blood results:

Na 137

K 4.9

Creatinine 100

eGFR 74

HBA1C 8.2% (previous 6 months ago was 7) or 55 mMol/mol

Total cholesterol 5.2 (previous was 4.2)

HDL 1.3

TGs 1.5

LDL 3.2

TC:HDL 4

ALT 54

Bilirubin 20

Alk Phos 140

Creatine Kinase 300

A6 Type 2 diabetes

Patient brief: Mr Steven James

You are a 54-year-old tablet-controlled diabetic who was diagnosed several years ago. Along with your diabetic medicine (metformin), which you take regularly twice a day, you also take a junior aspirin tablet to protect your heart once a day. You have not had any side effects from the medicine. If the doctor suggests you stop this you are concerned, as you have a strong family history of heart disease (mother and father both had heart attacks in their early 60s); you also used to smoke. However, if the doctor can convince you of the benefits of stopping the aspirin, you would follow their advice.

You would be happy to increase your diabetic tablet if advised accordingly, as it helped you lose weight when you first started it. You are, however, a little more sceptical about starting a cholesterol tablet, as your cholesterol has always been good and you have made strides to improve your diet as well as joining the gym. You are aware of what you should be doing to control your diabetes in terms of diet and exercise. You have recently been to a diabetes management group class that the nurse organised.

You only drink a small amount of alcohol socially. You have no problems taking the medicines, and have had no side effects. There are no problems in your personal life and work as an accountant is fine. You are single with no children.

Patient's opening remarks: *'Hello, doctor. The nurse asked me to come and see you about my diabetes.'*

Patient's agenda: You are wary of stopping your aspirin, but not closed to the possibility. If the doctor can explain why you should be on a cholesterol tablet then you would take it. If he or she suggests any new medicines then you would like to know about any potential side effects and when you should next come for a review or further tests.

EXAMINATION FINDINGS

If the candidate wishes to take a blood pressure reading, then they can (though it is not necessary). No other examination should be needed. BP: 130/72 today.

Reflection

Key points

- **Management:** This station revolves mainly around chronic disease management. After establishing that the patient has already made lifestyle changes to maximise diabetic control, you should now look at medications. Once any potential side effects and concordance problems have been disregarded, increasing the metformin would be sensible, as the HbA1C has risen significantly. A simple review of medication should prompt you to stop the aspirin, as the risks of bleeding outweigh any benefit here. Starting a statin, while explaining why it is necessary as well as any potential side effects, is key. Arrange a follow-up visit and blood tests.

Suggested marking criteria

	Clear Pass	Pass	Fail	Clear Fail
Data gathering	Social history, patient's fears over IHD given family history	Establishes concordance and side effects of medication	Does not enquire about concordance and any side effects of medication	Does not enquire about current lifestyle
Management	Arranges follow-up including bloods; stops aspirin	Starts a statin tablet, while explaining potential side effects	Increases metformin	No changes to medication
Interpersonal skills	Arranges follow-up bloods and review; explains the need for a statin effectively	Safety-netting, carefully deals with patient's concerns over IHD	Does not take into account what steps the patient has taken to change his lifestyle or his concerns over IHD	Didactic style of consulting; specifically delivery of information in a doctor-centred way

Trainer's comments

This patient has a worsening cholesterol and HbA1C despite adhering to a better diet with no significant weight change. Enquiring about the **patient's lifestyle** would reveal that he is quite motivated and fully aware of what he should be doing. The recent entry from the diabetic nurse, along with the revelation that he has recently been to a group diabetes class, should confirm this.

Given this, management of this chronic medical problem is the crux of this station. With the increase in HbA1C, the first step would be to check compliance and for any potential side effects of the medicine. Once you have established that there are no problems in either area, it would be best practice to **increase the metformin** dose to three times a day from twice a day.

You should explain that the latest evidence suggests that he ought to **stop his daily aspirin** due to risks of gastric bleeding, which, given there has not been a heart attack or stroke, outweighs any potential benefit, even with a 'non-significant' family history of cardiovascular disease (as both first-degree relatives were older than 60 when they had a cardiac event).

You should advise him to **start taking a statin** (as the patient is a diabetic over the age of 40). First-line choice would be simvastatin 40 mg once a day. The patient should be informed of the small chance of liver damage, which is monitored by a blood test at 3 and 12 months. There is also a small risk of muscle breakdown and damage. You should advise him to stop the statin if he gets symptoms of either complication. Explaining why a statin is useful for the patient but also explaining that the risks of aspirin outweigh the benefits is key to distinguishing between a pass and fail on management.

Safety-netting is important here. If the patient reports symptoms of rhabdomyolysis (weakness, muscle pain, darker urine), they must stop the statin and come in for a blood test. However, the tablets are very good at reducing cholesterol (which ought to be less than 4 for a diabetic), which at high levels is associated with heart disease.

You need to arrange blood tests for liver function, total cholesterol and HbA1C in 3 months, along with a **subsequent review** with a doctor or diabetic nurse. As there have been a lot of changes to medication here, check that the patient has a clear understanding of the plan if you have time.

Further Reading

Aspirin guidance from MHRA. http://www.mhra.gov.uk/Safetyinformation/DrugSafetyUpdate/CON087716

Barnett, H., Burrill, P. & Iheanacho, I. (2010) Don't use aspirin for primary prevention of cardiovascular disease. *British Medical Journal*, 340, c1805. http://www.bmj.com/content/340/bmj.c1805

National Institute for Health and Clinical Excellence (2009) *The Management of Type 2 Diabetes*. London: NICE. www.nice.org.uk/CG87

PATIENT

Name: Master James Wright

Age: 18 months (accompanied by his dad who is not registered at the practice)

SH: Nil

PMH: Nil

DH: Nil

Allergies: Penicillin

Immunisations: All up to date except second measles, mumps and rubella (MMR) booster due

Last consultation (GP notes):

Seen with mum, coryza last few days, temp, off food, no rash/vomiting/travel, regularly passing urine.

O/E Seen with mum. Appears well. Smells a bit. Unkempt.

Temp 37.7

HR 118

RR 24

Chest clear

ENT NAD

Warm peripheries

CRT < 2 sec

Hydrated; moist mucus membranes

Usual advice – see SOS 1/52 or vomiting/rash/lethargy/RR^

A7 Child protection

Patient brief: Father (Eric) to your son Master James Wright (18 months old)

You are a 35-year-old labourer and you are divorced from James's mother, Sharon Smith, who has a 7-year-old child from a different partner. As his biological father you have access to James at weekends. Recently you have been concerned about the mental health of your ex-partner (James's mother) as she seems 'down'. You have noticed that when he comes to stay with you he often smells as if he hasn't had a wash for a few days. You have also noticed that James has a few more bruises than usual, mainly on his legs. You put these down to him tripping over as he's getting used to walking.

You live alone with a long-term girlfriend. However, your ex-partner has a new boyfriend who was released from prison a few months ago. James stays at home with his mother, who is unemployed, and he attends a local nursery once a week; you could find out the details if required. This weekend your ex informed you that she was feeling a bit stressed, so she asked you to keep James for the next two weeks, which you're very happy to do. However, when you got home, you noticed that he had a new bruise on his ear. You are very concerned about this and have taken him to his GP for advice. You are not registered at the practice. You are not happy to return James to his mother in two weeks' time.

Patient's opening remarks: *'Doc, something's happened to my son, you've got to help.'*

Patient's agenda: You want to get to the bottom of who caused this bruise and are aware that this might involve the police and social services. You are concerned over your son's safety and are not keen on returning him to his mother, as you are worried he might be at risk of getting hurt again. You will only be satisfied if the doctor can convince you that this will be taken seriously and that the authorities will be involved swiftly.

EXAMINATION FINDINGS

The child has a small fresh but healing bruise to the ear and one on the shins.
No other bruises seen.
Fronulum intact.

Reflection
Key points
- **Data gathering:** Finding out who is at home with James and his mother and at the father's home is important. In addition, enquiring if James attends a nursery would be important to triangulate information, as well about his half-sister's school.

- **Management:** Red flags – same-day urgent social services referral, along with an attempt to measure the bruise for documentation.
- **Interpersonal skills:** Exploring the father's concerns thoroughly but sensitively could be one way to tackle this very sensitive case.

Suggested marking criteria

	Clear Pass	**Pass**	**Fail**	**Clear Fail**
Data gathering	Ascertains personal data of those in contact with James, as well as his nursery and half-sister's school; measures size of bruise	Ascertains social circumstances; how father thought the bruises got there; establishes that James attends nursery	Does not enquire over who lives with father	Does not enquire about home circumstances
Management	Arranges follow-up; mentions liaising with health visitors/ nursery/school; calls social services	Same-day urgent social services referral	Routine social services referral	No referral
Interpersonal skills	Is clear on the management plan	Takes a sensitive approach to a delicate topic; use of ICE	Fails to form rapport with father/(child)	Didactic style of consulting; specifically delivery of information in a doctor-centred way

Trainer's comments

To pass, you need to recognise that this is a **potentially serious child protection issue** and act appropriately. You need to ensure that the child is safe tonight. Given that the father is bringing in the child, it is likely that the child is safe with him for now, but you cannot assume that he is not involved.

In real life, **clear documentation** of the bruise and its size (ideally getting the father to take a picture) is good practice. **Same-day urgent referral** and a call to the social services child protection team are a must. This does not necessarily

mean that the child needs to go into care or to A&E today. However, your referral must be immediate so that social services can organise an urgent police visit to both parental homes, a same-week community paediatrician review, and an urgent child protection conference.

Referring to social services will need to be handled clearly and **sensitively**. The Pendleton 'ICE' (ideas, concerns and expectations) approach could help here (1); asking the father where he thought the bruises came from and what he thought should happen might be an effective way into the discussion. You should explain to him why you have to refer to social services: to find out what is going on and to ensure James's safety. Given the father's concerns, he is likely to accept this. Convincing him that things will be taken seriously and acted on swiftly should allay his fears and, if he asks, he should be advised to return his son to his mother as planned, otherwise he would be in trouble from the authorities. Social services would be making an urgent assessment into James's home circumstances to ensure his safety.

Exploring the parents' **home circumstances** and personal life is vital. Saying that you need James's mother's contact details (date of birth [DOB] and telephone number) is important, so that you can read her notes to help fill in the child protection referral form. You also need to know the father and his partner's address and DOB, so social services could look up their details (and, if relevant, the backgrounds of those living with them) to check whether they are known to them, or check with a different borough for child protection issues. Finding out which nursery James attends, and which school his half-sister attends, would also be helpful in order to gather some more objective information later on.

Make sure that you arrange **clear follow-up**, especially before James is due to be returned to his mother. It would be good to mention that you would also need to liaise with the local health visitors.

Reference

1. Pendleton, D., Schofield, T., Tate, P. & Havelock, P. (1984) *The Consultation: An Approach to Learning and Teaching*. Oxford: Oxford University Press.

Further Reading

RCGP Safeguarding Children Toolkit (2011) http://www.rcgp.org.uk/clinical-and-research/clinical-resources/child-and-adolescent-health/safeguarding-children-Toolkit/~/media/Files/CIRC/Safeguarding%20Children%20Module%20One/Safeguarding-Children-and-Young-People-Toolkit.ashx

Case A8

A8 Drug withdrawal

Patient brief: Mr Stan Beluski

You are a 28-year-old heroin user who has come to the doctor in desperation to try to give up. You also buy diazepam from the street and take 20–30 mg a day. You have been injecting 1 g of heroin since you turned 25. This coincided with you losing your job for repeatedly turning up late having partied too much the night before.

You are from Poland and moved here to look for work, as things back home were bad. Your father was an alcoholic and used to beat you and your mother. You are an only child and used to self-harm as a teenager when you were very depressed, but you haven't felt that low or suicidal for years. Your father died several years ago and as there were limited opportunities in Poland, you moved to the UK to look for work. You met your ex-partner and have a 2-year-old child together, but after you turned to drugs to cope with your unemployment and low mood, she moved out and you only fleetingly see your daughter in your ex's company.

You moved to the area a month ago to live with a friend who is not on drugs, with the aim of avoiding bumping into your previous associates who use drugs. You have never really wanted to give up as much as you do now. You have been considering this for a month. You have stolen cars to fund your drug habit and although you have never been caught, you want to give up this lifestyle to get on the 'straight and narrow'.

You last 'scored' more than 24 hours ago and you are starting to feel the effects of not having the drug. You are feeling very nauseous, sweating and panicky. You have enough diazepam for the weekend.

Patient's opening remarks: '*Look doctor, I'm in a bad way and I really need your help here…*'

Patient's agenda: You would be willing to engage with a specialist drug rehab team, but you're aware that it is Friday evening and they won't be open until Monday. You just need something to get you through the weekend. You have not gone more than 24 hours without heroin for years, and you're worried that if you do not get something from the doctor tonight, you will have to go back onto drugs, which is something you really do not want to do. You will need to push the doctor on this.

EXAMINATION FINDINGS

Pulse 118 regular
Sweating
Pupils normal size
BP 100/78
Afebrile

Reflection
Key points
- **Management:** Candidates should not prescribe any drugs to combat opiate withdrawal, but should refer to the local drug rehabilitation team. Consider anti-emetics only to help combat nausea.

- **Interpersonal skills:** The key skill is forming rapport and congratulating the patient on trying to give up. An acceptable plan should also be negotiated for both of you. It is important to enquire about home circumstances and any children at home.

Suggested marking criteria

	Clear Pass	Pass	Fail	Clear Fail
Data gathering	Explores past childhood and forensic history	Social circumstances and mood explored	No home circumstances enquired about; does not explore mood	Does not enquire about method or amount of drug use
Management	Arranges follow-up; prescribes anti-emetics	Refuses to prescribe opiates and refers to local drug rehab team	Prescribes weak opiates to combat effects	Prescribes methadone, diazepam or buprenorphine
Interpersonal skills	Is firm but kind in refusal to prescribe	Empathetic approach	Fails to form rapport	Didactic style of consulting; specifically delivery of information in a doctor-centred way

Trainer's comments

There's an important **red flag** here. Prescriptions from drug rehab teams can be signed by most GPs, but initiating opiate withdrawal or maintenance treatment is a specialist field within primary care. The worry here is that without a urine sample confirming opiates in the bloodstream, starting to give methadone or buprenorphine (brand name Subutex; medicines used to help treat opiate addiction) to an opiate-naïve patient could result in respiratory arrest. Likewise, 30 mg of diazepam taken as a one-off dose could have the same effect.

It is important to try to be **understanding and non-judgemental** in this situation; make it clear that you want to help, that you will be making an urgent referral to the local drug rehabilitation team, and that you can offer medication to help with the sickness. An **empathetic but firm refusal** to prescribe any opiates is the appropriate response here. Patients may be quite aggressive and threaten to do many things to avoid opiate withdrawal, but this will not kill them, while your prescription pad could. A reasonable response to repeated, desperate requests of '*What will I do until next week*?' could be 'Well, you need to do what you have to to manage.'

It would help to get some background to the patient's past and to **build rapport** so that you can form a therapeutic doctor–patient relationship for the future. **Congratulate the patient** for wanting to come off opiates, but explain that this needs to be planned with the input of a **local drug rehabilitation team**. They would send his urine off to a laboratory to confirm opiate addiction (some do have bedside urine dipsticks for this purpose). Patients are often started on low doses of methadone (for example, 30 ml daily) with daily review and slow gradual increases of dose (5 ml) until there are no withdrawal symptoms. This is done in shared care with a local pharmacist who can dispense daily pick-ups and ideally has facilities for supervised consumption. Patients will often use heroin on top of this, which is a risk.

You should try to establish whether the patient has ever been in trouble with the police and who they are living with at home. Don't forget any potential **child protection** issues, but this patient does not have any unsupervised time with his child.

Finding out what drugs he takes, and how, is important. Referring to the local drug rehabilitation team and ensuring **follow-up** in the practice would be a minimum. It would be good to try to prescribe something for the **nausea** (simple anti-emetic), but not any other opiates (like dihydrocodeine) or benzodiazepines.

For women, it may be prudent at times to discuss contraception and cytological screening; and for those injecting, **needle advice**. It can be important to enquire about blood-borne virus testing (HIV/hepatitis) in those injecting as well as offering to check injecting sites for infection.

Further Reading

Royal College of General Practitioners (2011) Guidance for the use of substitute prescribing in the treatment of opioid dependence in primary care. http://www.smmgp.org.uk/download/guidance/guidance004.pdf

Case A9

PATIENT

Name: Miss Stefanie Small (brought in by her mother)
Age: 6 years 3 months
PMH: Eczema, asthma
DH: Salbutamol, aqueous cream, hydrocortisone cream

Last consultation (1 week ago):
Seen by practice nurse
Asthma review
Symptoms stable, RCP questions 0; moderate inhaler technique; never smoked;
PEFR 200 Needs blue inhaler a few times a week
Eczema: flare-up, non-infected – start steroid cream, side effects warned, see SOS

A9 Paediatric eczema

Patient brief: Mother (Sarah) of Miss Stefanie Small (6-year-old child)

You are a 38-year-old single secretary. You have brought your 6-year-old daughter to the GP to try to sort out her eczema. She was diagnosed a couple of years ago and you have tried a few moisturising creams (aqueous cream and E45) to no avail. Stefanie (your daughter) also has mild asthma, but that is fine and the practice nurse did a check last time. However, the eczema on her hands is no better and you demand to see a dermatologist or an allergy doctor, as you fear she is allergic to something. This was triggered by something you read on an internet forum for mothers.

There is a family history of hayfever only. If asked, you have not been that compliant with the moisturising cream and you bathe Stefanie in normal soaps. You did use the steroid cream, but not with much aqueous cream.

Everything else in Stefanie's life is fine, both at school and at home. If asked why you have not been compliant with her creams, you will explain that your time is short as you have to juggle a part-time job and looking after her. You have no extra support. However, if the doctor can prescribe double the amount of medication, you could get the school nurse to administer one dose of creams, and that would reduce the burden for you.

You are fine in yourself and not stressed or low. You have not noticed that any particular food substances trigger her eczema.

Patient's opening remarks: '*It's taken me so long to get a follow-up appointment; I really want Stefanie seen by a specialist…*'

Patient's agenda: You are worried about her diagnosis and that the treatment is not working. You think she may be allergic to something. You want to see a

---

specialist. But if the doctor can convince you how to use the creams correctly and what to avoid, as well as offer you a clear management plan, then you would back off from demanding a referral. You have not used the steroid cream that much since you saw the last GP, as you have some concerns over their side effects, but again, if the doctor can explain why you need to use it you will.

EXAMINATION FINDINGS

If asked, Stefanie's hands show only mild non-infected eczema.

Reflection

Key points

- **Interpersonal skills:** It is important to find out details of home and school life in the context of a child with a chronic illness that is not resolving. Once it is established that there is a difficulty complying with the creams, exploring the reasons behind this would help build rapport and allow the patient to consider sharing solutions.

Replying to referral requests with an immediate 'no' can cause conflict, so perhaps consider alternative responses that you can practise (there is detailed feedback in the trainer's comments).

Giving a clear explanation of the diagnosis and management plan (including side effects of medication and ways to combat them) and ensuring there is adequate follow-up will also help deal with the situation.

Suggested marking criteria

	Clear Pass	Pass	Fail	Clear Fail
Data gathering	Elicits why the patient wants to be referred	Explores compliance with medication and social circumstances	Does not enquire about home circumstances	Does not explore use of medication
Management	Arranges follow-up; comes up with solution to cope with poor compliance	Gives a clear management plan for how to apply medications	Increases the dose of steroid cream	Refers on to specialist
Interpersonal skills	Deals with referral request adequately	Uses non-jargon to explain diagnosis and management plan	Fails to form rapport or be empathetic to circumstances	Didactic style of consulting; specifically delivery of information in a doctor-centred way

Trainer's comments

Exploring who is at home and what is going on at school is important whenever you consult about a child. As the child is technically not present, you will need to improvise. Asking about **compliance** and Stefanie's bathing routine will reveal poor concordance, but you should explore any reasons for this in a **non-judgemental** fashion. Once you have established that Stefanie's mother is too busy to administer her creams, you could empathise with her and then go on to discuss some **practical solutions**. Asking the mother what might help her could generate some useful ideas (for example, doubling the amount you give on prescriptions, so that the school can also administer). Remember, we do not have as much insight into our patients' lives as they do.

This station tests your skills in dealing with **demanding patients**. When faced with an opening gambit of '*I want a referral*' or '*I want this medication*', instead of saying 'no', which can often trigger immediate and unhelpful conflict, there are various ways of saying 'yes… but no'. An example here might be: 'Yes, of course we can refer her, if that's necessary; now tell me in a bit more detail what's going on.' This does not commit you to a referral, but gets you out of a potentially sticky situation trying to balance the patient's expectations with your gate-keeping role.

Referring straightforward contact dermatitis or eczema in an otherwise well child who has no features of allergy (i.e. a regular obvious trigger for symptoms that are widespread or associated with non-skin symptoms, like diarrhoea) would not be the best use of scarce NHS resources. You could also point out to the mother that she might have to take time off work to attend frequent hospital appointments. It would be far better for the GP to **manage the eczema properly together with the mother**, before referring on if it is not improving.

Sometimes, you may need the help of a dermatology nurse specialist to help with advice over administering creams, but that could be done later. Reassuring the mother that if you (pleural 'you' here – the problem is shared between you, the mother and the child) are not making progress with the condition, then you would **plan to refer**, might help allay any fears.

Establishing a washing and moisturising regime is likely to reveal some areas of practice that could be improved. For example, aqueous cream is irritant to eczematous skin when used as a moisturising cream, but is useful as a soap substitute (i.e. washed off after application). The evidence for using bath additives is limited, but for clear-cut contact dermatitis of the hands, aqueous cream could be helpful. Liberal use of a medicated moisturising cream (such as diprobase or doublebase) is the next step, followed by a mild **topical steroid** approximately 30 minutes later.

It is important to explain the rationale for using steroid creams or ointments (effective treatment of flare-ups), but to warn the parent of the potential side effects of prolonged use of steroid creams (skin thinning). Explain that to reduce that risk they should only use them for a **limited period** (for example, up to 2 weeks). Being clear and confident with the diagnosis and management plan can reduce the parent's concerns and fears. Ensuring follow-up soon would also help.

Further Reading

National Institute for Health and Clinical Excellence (2007) *Atopic Eczema in Children: Management of Atopic Eczema in Children from Birth up to the Age of 12 years*. London: NICE. http://guidance.nice.org.uk/CG57

Case A10 📷

A10 Renal colic

Patient brief: Mr Anil Mukerjee

You are a 38-year-old lawyer who runs his own successful firm. You have made an emergency appointment to see the doctor today, as you have had the most awful pain in your stomach you could ever have imagined. It was severe, sharp and, if asked, rated at 10/10. You had to take paracetamol and ibuprofen, which didn't do much. It lasted a few hours and came in waves. Nothing triggered it off. If asked, it was around the right side of your stomach and spread on that side down to your groin. If asked, you felt nauseous but did not vomit. You have had no problems with urinating or opening your bowels and have not seen blood in either. You have not had a temperature.

Things are stressful and busy at work, but you are coping fine. Sleep isn't great, as you have a 4-month-old baby, but you are overjoyed at fatherhood. You realise you haven't been terribly supportive at home, as you are not around as much you could be. You are considering hiring a nanny to help your wife. You do not have any major medical problems or any significant family medical history, apart from diabetes (your father in his 60s).

Your diet of late has been poor, with lots of takeaway food. In addition, to combat the lack of sleep, you have turned to regular cups of coffee (more than 10 cups a day). Your mood is fine.

Patient's opening remarks: *'I've had this really terrible stomach pain, doctor, and paracetamol just doesn't touch it.'*

Patient's agenda: The pain is easing now, but you would like to know what it was and, if it came again, what stronger painkillers you could take. If the doctor suggests you go to hospital, even if they explain the importance of this, you cannot afford to leave today as you run your own business. However, if a planned appointment could be made then you could rearrange work commitments.

EXAMINATION FINDINGS

Abdo exam: soft, non-tender, no rebound/guarding/peritonism. BS present. No hernia. Normal testes.

If asked:
HR 92
BP 134/84
Temp 37C
Urine dipstick: 2+ blood

Reflection
Key points
- **Data gathering:** Important to form a working diagnosis of renal colic by ruling out more urgent differential diagnoses (appendicitis, testicular torsion, obstructing hernia, abdominal aortic aneurysm, urinary tract infection [UTI]). This can be done with a focused history (no fever, vomiting, bowels open, not a smoker, no urinary symptoms) and backed up with a normal examination.
- **Management:** If urgent investigations cannot be arranged, then the patient should go to A&E. However, once it becomes clear he cannot attend A&E, being flexible should prompt you to arrange urgent investigations yourself. Assess renal function that day (BP, urine dipstick and eGFR blood test) and arrange an urgent CT scan of the kidneys, ureters and bladder (CT KUB) within a week. As a safety-net, explain that he should hear from the hospital about a scan within a week, but that if he gets the pain again, has a fever or becomes unwell, he should present again.
- **Interpersonal skills:** Exploring his social history, forming rapport and ensuring that he is aware that he can access help from the surgery if needed are probably the important aspects in this station.

Suggested marking criteria

	Clear Pass	Pass	Fail	Clear Fail
Data gathering	Explore why the patient is too busy at home/work	Rules out urgent differential diagnosis	Completes abdomenal exam including urine dipstick and BP	No history of fever, vomiting or questions to rule out a significant differential diagnosis
Management	Lifestyle advice; safety-netting	Arranges same-day bloods and CT KUB within a week	Refers to A&E without regard for patient circumstances	Simple analgesia
Interpersonal skills	Deals with home/work situation sensitively	Uses non-jargon to explain diagnosis and management plan; elicits ICE	Fails to form rapport or be empathetic to circumstances	Didactic style of consulting; specifically delivery of information in a doctor-centred way

Trainer's comments

Ruling out the absolute need for hospital admission is paramount. You need to form a working **diagnosis of renal colic** and rule out more **urgent differential diagnoses** (appendicitis, testicular torsion, obstructing hernia, abdominal aortic aneurysm [AAA], UTI). This can be done with a focused history (no fever, vomiting, bowels open, not a smoker, no urinary symptoms) and backed up with a normal examination. Given that the patient's pain is improving and he has no vomiting or fever, he could be **managed safely within general practice**.

The diagnosis can be made on the **classic history** and the **urine dipstick**, but remember that a small but significant proportion of renal colic patients will *not* have microscopic haematuria.

Then the focus should be a clear and appropriate management plan, along with tight safety-netting. It could be argued that if you can't arrange urgent investigations, then the patient should go to A&E. However, once it becomes clear that he cannot attend A&E, you should be flexible enough to **arrange investigations yourself from the surgery**. The first part is to assess renal function that day (BP, urine dipstick and eGFR blood test). Remember that even if your practice does not have in-house phlebotomy, you could take the patient's blood or even ask him to attend the hospital for this, as it is likely to be quicker than A&E. The next part would be to arrange a CT KUB scan within a week. You would need to explain to the patient that you have to call the CT department to order this test, and that you would need to check the patient's contact details so that the appointment could be phoned through.

Safety-netting is very important in this case. This means explaining that the patient should expect to hear from the hospital about a scan within a week, but that if they get the pain again, have a fever or become unwell, they should present again. In the interim, ensure that the patient has **adequate pain relief** (NSAIDs, paracetamol, codeine) and drinks plenty of water.

This patient is not depressed and is coping; he has already devised a plan to try to alleviate the pressure on his partner at home. Exploring what is going on at work and why the patient cannot take time off to deal with an illness will help build **rapport** and allow you to better understand what is going on at home.

Further Reading

Bultitude, M. & Rees, J. (2012) Management of renal colic. *British Medical Journal*, 345, 30–35. http://www.bmj.com/content/345/bmj.e5499

Case A11 🎥

PATIENT

Name: Ms Pauline Withers
Age: 42
SH: Ex-smoker
PMH: Hyperthyroidism, OA knee (current problems); anxiety and depression (past problem, inactive for 10 years)
DH: Co-codamol 8/500; ibuprofen gel; carbimazole 5 mg

A11 Upper respiratory tract infection

Patient brief: Ms Pauline Withers

You are a busy 42-year-old head teacher at a local school. You have had a sore throat for the past 2 days. There has been no temperature, rash or vomiting. You have had a mild cough and a slight headache with no other symptoms. You have not been abroad recently, but would like some antibiotics for this illness. If asked, you last had a throat infection a few years ago and the doctor then told you it was 'just a virus'. But a week later you were no better and had to take a week off work to recuperate. You needed to go to hospital then and they gave you antibiotics, which worked. You understand that antibiotics do not work for viral illnesses and if the doctor can placate and reason with you, you will reveal that this illness does not feel as bad as the last one. If the doctor can explain why this one is more likely to be caused by a virus, then you would be willing to accept their explanation. However, you are aware that things could get worse, and you cannot afford to take time off work to attend again or to stay at home and recover.

You have an OFSTED inspection visit next week and have lots of paperwork that needs to be filled in and teachers to be chased. You are understandably stressed with this but are not down, and once this is over you will have your summer holidays to look forward to. You are single and, if asked, in the past suffered with depression after your parents passed away. You take a painkiller for your arthritic knee and a tablet for an overactive thyroid, which was diagnosed last year. You had your annual hospital clinic review last month, where they checked your thyroid blood levels and you were told all was fine. They are seeing you again in 6 months. You are an ex-smoker and drink socially only.

If the doctor wants to arrange a blood test today for you, you kick up a fuss and explain you only had one last month and were told all was fine. If the doctor insists, then you will do one, but only after the OFSTED visit next week. However, if the doctor can explain clearly why the test needs to be done today, then you will attend the hospital/practice and get it done.

Patient's opening remarks: *'I've come about my throat – I'm not feeling very well at all and I think I really need some antibiotics for it.'*

Patient's agenda: You are very busy with an imminent OFSTED inspection and you can't afford to take time off. Because antibiotics worked last time, you think that's what you really need this time. But you can be persuaded that it might not be necessary this time and that you need a blood test today (if doctor explains clearly the risks).

EXAMINATION FINDINGS

The candidate should be free to examine this patient as they see fit. Ideally:

HR
BP
Throat
Lymph nodes
Chest exam

All should be **normal,** like the fictitious patient.

Reflection

Key points

- **Management:** Red flags – it's important to arrange same-day FBC to rule out bone-marrow suppression as the patient is on carbimazole. CENTOR criteria (1) are clear that antibiotics are not indicated in this case. However, the use of delayed antibiotics would avoid the need for this patient to take time off work to return for treatment. As a safety-net, ensure the patient knows to seek medical attention if she has difficulty swallowing, breathing or develops a rash; and make sure the patient's contact details are correct.

- **Interpersonal skills:** Exploring the personal circumstances of the patient and recognising that she is very busy and stressed will make managing this case easier.

Suggested marking criteria

	Clear Pass	Pass	Fail	Clear Fail
Data gathering	Elicits concerns over work; explores stresses	Adequate physical examination	Elicits no fever/rash/ vomiting/ allergies but cough present	No history of fever, vomiting or questions to rule out a significant differential diagnoses
Management	Negotiates delayed prescription of antibiotics	Arranges same-day FBC, safety-netting	No same-day blood test arranged	Prescribes antibiotics from today
Interpersonal skills	Gives options for treatment (no antibiotics v delayed)	Uses non-jargon to explain diagnosis and management plan; elicits ICE	Fails to form rapport or be empathetic to circumstances	Didactic style of consulting; specifically delivery of information in a doctor-centred way

Trainer's comments

Patients on potentially bone-marrow suppressant drugs like carbimazole, mirtazapine or lamotrogine need to have an **urgent same-day full blood count** performed if they present with symptoms of agranulocytosis (sore throat, fever, bruising, malaise, mouth ulcers or a non-specific illness). Ideally, the patient should be told this on starting the medication, but it is the doctor's responsibility to arrange this. This test could be done in practice (and sent to hospital urgently), in hospital phlebotomy (but marked urgent) or, if it's not possible to get the results back that day (for example, out of hours or late afternoon), then in A&E.

Exploring the **personal circumstances** of the patient and recognising that she is very busy and stressed will aid your management. It would be good practice to explore her work and personal life and offer support; but in this case the patient is likely to decline it.

You should try to explore **what the patient thinks** may be going on and what she is worried about, as well as what she might want; this makes it much more likely that she will accept your management suggestions. Once you have established that the patient is concerned about getting as ill as before, you could explain that she does not have the features of the bacterial illness she had last time, but that she could access treatment quickly if needed.

While antibiotics are not indicated in this case, evidence from the Drug and Therapeutics Bulletin and NICE suggests the use of delayed antibiotics, which would avoid the need for this patient to take time off work for future treatment [2, 3]. Giving the patient the option of **no treatment or delayed antibiotics** (and when to take them) would be good practice. A delayed prescription for 10 days of phenoxymethylpenicillin 500 mg QDS could be issued, checking for penicillin allergy.

References

1. Centor, R.M., Witherspoon, J.M., Dalton, H.P., Brody, C.E. & Link, K. (1981) The diagnosis of strep throat in adults in the emergency room. *Medical Decision Making*, 1 (3): 239–246. PMID 6763125
2. National Institute for Health and Clinical Excellence (NICE) (2008) *Self-Limiting Respiratory Tract Infections in Adults and Children in Primary Care*. London: NICE. http://www.nice.org.uk/CG69
3. Tan, T., Little, P. & Stokes, T.; Guideline Development Group (2008) Antibiotic prescribing for self limiting respiratory tract infections in primary care: Summary of NICE guidance. *British Medical Journal*, 337: a437. http://www.bmj.com/content/337/bmj.a437

Further Reading

Little, P., Moore, M. & Williamson, I. (2009) Effect of antibiotic prescribing strategies and an information leaflet on longer-term reconsultation for acute lower respiratory tract infection. *British Journal of General Practice*, 59 (567): 728–734. doi: 10.3399/bjgp09X472601

Case A12 🖾

PATIENT

Setting: The district nurse has asked you to visit the next patient at home. She feels the patient has been getting more breathless over the past few days and may not be coping at home.

Name: Mrs Annie Frith

Age: 77

PMH: Breast cancer (T3N2M1) with metastases to liver and chest
　　　　Moderate aortic stenosis
　　　　High cholesterol
　　　　Hypertension
　　　　Osteoarthritis of the knee
　　　　Osteoporosis
　　　　Diverticulitis
　　　　Hysterectomy (40 years ago)

DH: Paracetamol 1 g qds
　　　Alendronic acid 70 mg weekly
　　　Adcal D3 2 T
　　　Bendroflumethiazide 2.5 mg
　　　Topical ibuprofen
　　　Simvastatin 40 mg nocte

Last consultation (by GP, 10 days ago):
　　　Home visit:
　　　Discussion about diagnosis, aware of poor prognosis.
　　　Not in pain currently.
　　　No relatives.
　　　Coping but may need input.
　　　Completed palliative chemo; not for active treatment.
　　　District nurse to visit to help administer medication.
　　　Meals on Wheels arranged. Social services referral sent.

A12 Palliative care

Patient brief: Mrs Annie Frith

You are a 77-year-old widow who has terminal breast cancer that has spread to your lungs and liver. Last month you completed some chemotherapy, but this was to reduce your breathlessness. It did work, but you would not want to go through that again as it made you feel so sick. You live alone, having survived your husband, who passed away from a heart attack a few years ago. You have no children and were an only child. Any distant relatives live in Ireland and you are not in touch. You have a friendly neighbour who lives close by, but they are abroad at the moment.

You have become more breathless in the last week and have been experiencing a sharp pain in the upper right part of your abdomen, where the cancer spread. You think that is where your liver is; at least, that is what the cancer specialist told you. You have been experiencing the pain for several weeks and it is starting to become more unbearable.

You are eating and drinking, but find it difficult to take lots of tablets. You are happy to take some, especially painkillers. You are aware that the district nurse has called the doctor out as you are in more pain and are more breathless than usual.

Patient's opening remarks: *'I'm just feeling really breathless and I've got pain in my tummy here…'*

Patient's agenda: If suggested, you do not want to go to hospital or a hospice. You wish to die in your flat, as it is where you grew up and it holds fond memories of your husband. You are prepared to die and are at one with God. You are a devout Christian and have called the local minister, who will be arriving later to pray with you. You are a bit scared of dying alone, but this would not make you leave your home. If asked, you are happy not to be resuscitated and are willing to be seen by the palliative care team, whom you met once on the ward.

EXAMINATION FINDINGS

Chest exam unremarkable but RR22 HR 100 BP 128/68

Abdominal exam: soft tender right upper quadrant no rebound/guarding/peritonism. BS present

If asked sats 90% room air

Reflection

Key points

- **Data gathering:** Examining the chest and taking the oxygen saturations should prompt the candidate to recognise the need to order palliative oxygen.
- **Interpersonal skills:** It's important to explore the patient's fear of dying alone and any spiritual needs she may have. Explain that towards the final stages of the illness, a Marie Curie nurse (or equivalent) could be arranged to come and sit with her.

- **Management:** You should support her as much as possible in her wish to die at home: for example, by referring her to the palliative care team and providing symptomatic relief. This would consist of analgesia and oxygen. Insisting that the patient go to hospital would be inappropriate. It is worth having a frank but sensitive discussion regarding her resuscitation status. While the patient is still able to swallow there is no need to start syringe drivers, but it might help to explain that some medicines could be stopped to reduce the oral burden.

Suggested marking criteria

	Clear pass	Pass	Fail	Clear Fail
Data gathering	Explores what has been discussed about end-of-life care wishes before	Establishes need for analgesia and reducing oral burden	Fails to examine the patient	Fails to elicit where she wants to die
Management	Prescribes palliative oxygen, considers hospice as an option, considers side effects of analgesia	Reduces oral medicines, discussion over resuscitation status	Refers to palliative care team alone; starts analgesia with no regard to side effects	Insists on referral to A&E or hospital
Interpersonal skills	Explores fears of dying alone	Empathetic and sensitive discussion over end-of-life needs	Fails to form rapport or be empathetic to circumstances	Fails to listen to patient's wishes

Trainer's comments

Examining the chest and taking the oxygen saturations should prompt you to recognise the need to order palliative oxygen. This can be ordered via a HOOF (Home Oxygen Order Form). Insisting

that the patient goes to hospital would be inappropriate.

Exploring the patient's fear of dying alone and any spiritual needs she may have (simply signposting them or asking the palliative care team to arrange a visit by her local spiritual leader) would be important.

You could try offering support via a hospice, but once it is clear that the patient wants to die at home, you should do what you can to support her decision. Referring to the palliative care team is part of this, but so is symptomatic relief. This would consist of analgesia (oral weak opiates to start, then morphine-based analgesia, not forgetting to co-prescribe medication to combat the side effects) and oxygen as above.

If time allows, stopping some unnecessary medication (bendroflumethazide, simvastatin) to reduce the oral burden might be prudent.

Further Reading

RCGP. End of life care resources for GPs. http://www.rcgp.org.uk/endoflife care

Case A13 📹

Name: Mrs Anne Maguire
Age: 42
PMH: Vitreous detachment R eye 5 years ago; eczema; hayfever
DH: Nil

A13 Acute stress

Patient brief: Mrs Annie Maguire

You are a 42-year-old receptionist. You have been feeling down for the past couple of months. Your husband, David, was diagnosed with terminal lung cancer 6 months ago and you are aware that he doesn't have long to live. You have three children (aged 20, 18 and 14) who all live at home; they are understandably upset, but coping. You are not sleeping well and although you enjoy your time with your husband, you cannot seem to stop crying.

This has become embarrassing at work, to such an extent that you have had to take the last week off. Your boss is aware of what is going on, but said that you would need a sick note if you were going to take longer off. Work is supportive. If asked, although it would be nice to be off work and spend more time with your husband, you are worried over finances and are keen not to lose too much income by being off sick long term; and you are also concerned about having a poor illness record. Your job involves face-to-face client interaction in busy large estate agents. If asked, you are aware of back-office work that involves less face-to-face customer interaction, and if the doctor suggests something like this, you would be willing to try it.

You have some close friends who are supportive. You are tired and have little energy at times, but do enjoy your time with your husband. You drink socially only and have never smoked. Apart from an eye problem once (you have no symptoms at the moment), you don't really have any medical problems (bar seasonal hayfever and occasional dry skin). You have never felt this way before. If asked, you occasionally think *'What's the point in carrying on with life?'* but have never made any plans to harm yourself, as you love your children too much and it would also belittle what David is going through.

Patient's opening remarks: '*I'm having a really hard time and I'm feeling tired and overwhelmed. I just wondered if there was anything I could have to help me with my energy*.'

Patient's agenda: If asked, you would like something to help you sleep. You don't really have time for counselling, but may consider it at a later date. You wonder if there is any medicine or 'tonic' that can make you feel a little better or give you more energy. You are worried about taking too much time off work.

EXAMINATION FINDINGS

No interaction.

If asked for a PHQ9 score, say you do not have that information but the candidate can perform one if they feel the need.

Reflection

Key points

- **Data gathering:** Recognising that this patient is going through an acute stress response and not clinical depression is key. You should ask about deliberate self-harm (DSH) as an assessment of risk.

- **Management:** Prescribing an antidepressant would be poor practice on this first visit to the doctor. A fit note would help manage work issues, and arranging follow-up would be good practice. Starting sleeping tablets would be poor practice, unless you explained that this would be to correct her sleep cycle and that this would be a one-off short supply. Explaining sleep hygiene, the use of self-help books, exercise, friends who listen or internet-based CBT could all be options avoiding the need for medication.

- **Interpersonal skills:** Exploring work circumstances, as well as support both at home and at work, would be important. Finding out the ages of children and how they are coping is also key.

Suggested marking criteria

	Clear Pass	Pass	Fail	Clear Fail
Data gathering	Explores home and work situation	DSH, acute stress response symptoms	Fails to ask about deliberate self-harm	Fails to enquire about children and their ages
Management	Self-help books, emergency contact details; Macmillan nurses	Fit note, sleep hygiene	Prescribes an inappropriate amount of sleeping tablets or fails to explain their addictive nature	Prescribes an antidepressant
Interpersonal skills	Tackles request for medication sensitively but responsibly	Empathetic and sensitive discussion over problems and ways to help	Fails to form rapport or be empathetic to circumstances	Fails to listen to patient's wishes

Trainer's comments

Recognising that this patient is going through an acute stress response and **not clinical depression** is key. Performing a Patient Health Questionnaire-9 (PHQ9) would reveal a high score, but this would be natural and normal in this circumstance. Prescribing an antidepressant would be poor practice on this first visit to the doctor. However, it is imperative that you ask about deliberate self-harm as an assessment of risk.

You should explore work circumstances, as well as **support both at home and work**. Find out the ages of the children and how they are coping too. This shows genuine interest in her situation, as well as giving you important contextual information.

In terms of management, you could try offering counselling, but once it becomes clear that the patient has too much on to attend, you should swiftly move on. A **fit note** suggesting 'avoiding face-to-face client interaction' temporarily might help to manage work issues, and arranging follow-up with you would be good practice.

Tackling the request for medication needs to be handled sensitively. Starting **sleeping tablets** would be poor practice, unless you explained the long-term risks and that this would be to correct her sleep cycle in the very short term so you would only give a very small supply. Explaining **sleep hygiene**, the use of self-help books, exercise, friends who listen and internet-based CBT (for example, Mood Gym (1) could all be options that would avoid the need for medication. Don't forget that repeat visits to the doctor could also help in the form of limited psychological therapy (2). Offering emergency contact details should the patient feel suicidal would be good practice. Signposting her to Macmillan nurses who can support relatives and carers would also be a good idea.

References

1. Mood Gym, http://www.moodgym. anu.edu.au
2. Balint, M. (2000) *The Doctor, His Patient and the Illness*. Millennium edn. Edinburgh: Churchill Livingstone.

Further Reading

National Institute for Health and Clinical Excellence (NICE) (2009) *Depression: The Treatment and Management of Depression in Adults (update)*. London: NICE. http://www.nice.org.uk/guidance/index.jsp?action=byID&o=12329

Cases (B)

How to Pass the CSA Exam, First Edition. Imtiaz Ahmad, Raj Nair, Martin Block and Graham Easton.
© 2015 John Wiley & Sons, Ltd. Published 2015 by John Wiley & Sons, Ltd.

Case B1 📃

PATIENT

Name: Ms Jane Dibble
Age: 27
SH: Smokes 10 cigarettes/day; alcohol occasionally (max 4 drinks/week)
PMH: Nil of note
DH: No current medication

B1 Irritable bowel syndrome

Patient brief: Ms Jane Dibble

You are a 27-year-old accountant who has had central abdominal pain and bloating, which is worse on eating, for the past 6 months.

Recently your stools have been intermittently loose, then hard, and you have been opening your bowels more often than is normal for you (two or three times a day instead of once). Your pain improves on opening your bowels. There is no blood or mucus in your stool and you are occasionally nauseous but have not vomited.

If asked, you do not have any vaginal discharge or pain on intercourse. You have no urinary symptoms. Your periods are sometimes irregular where the cycle has been occasionally longer or shorter than normal (28 days usually). Your last period was 2 weeks ago. You have been using condoms with your partner.

You have been highly stressed due to work overload at this time of year and you have an unsupportive partner who is '*always busy watching sport on TV*'.

Your mother died of breast cancer and you are worried because she complained of being bloated for years. You've read that bloating can be a dangerous sign for conditions such as ovarian cancer. You enjoy spicy foods and have been eating more takeaways recently so have actually gained weight, if asked. You drink alcohol socially but never more than four drinks and you smoke ten cigarettes a day. You don't find time to do regular exercise.

Patient's opening remarks: '*I've just come in because I keep getting uncomfortable in my tummy – I keep getting bloated and stuff*.'

Patient's agenda: You would like to know possible causes of your pain and start treatment for it today. You are worried that it might be something serious like ovarian cancer.

EXAMINATION FINDINGS

Abdominal exam: soft, mild central tenderness, no rebound or guarding. BS normal

PR (if offered with chaperone) NAD

BP 124/74

HR 76 Reg

Urinalysis NAD

Pregnancy test negative (if asked for)

Reflection

Key points

- **Data gathering:** It's important to cover appropriate examination and investigations. You need to exclude red flags such as pregnancy, STDs, urinary tract infections, appendicitis, malignancy (for example, ovarian cancer).

- **Management:** Adopt an evidence-based approach to diagnosing and managing irritable bowel syndrome. Try to address stress management. Remember the ethical dimension of NHS rationing and not sending for a 2-week-wait cancer referral.

- **Interpersonal skills:** This is a stressed but confident woman who is worried about her abdominal pains. She is a good historian, but is challenging about any vague diagnosis for her symptoms. It is important here to explore the patient's health beliefs about bloating and its link to cancer, as well as stress at home/work and an unsupportive partner. Be aware of patient autonomy and respect for confidentiality.

Suggested marking criteria

	Clear Pass	Pass	Fail	Clear Fail
Data gathering	Addresses differentials of abdominal pain; social history reviewed, including strain on relationship	Social history reviewed; limited discussion around differentials; checks that is not pregnant	No exclusion of red flag differentials; limited social history established	No exclusion of red flags; no social history or discussion around diagnosis or management
Management	Correct examination and clear discussion of management options	Medication prescribed with majority of advice; simple blood tests (FBC, CRP, ESR, coeliac, autoAbs)	Medication given without advice or follow-up	No advice or medication given; extensive investigation or 2-week-wait referral
Interpersonal skills	Establishes health beliefs, delivers information in bite-size chunks and summarises at the end	Establishes health beliefs and picks up cues; non-judgemental in consulting style	Fails to pick up cues, e.g. worries over malignancies, stress at home/work	Didactic style of consulting with no emotion shown towards the patient

Trainer's comments

You should be able to make a **positive diagnosis** of irritable bowel syndrome (IBS) in this patient, and confidently manage her in general practice. She exhibits typical features of IBS (6 months of abdominal pain discomfort, bloating and change in bowel habit).

It is important to listen to her story and then probe further with closed questions. These need to **exclude** urinary or gynaecological causes (checking last menstrual period and excluding pregnancy) and also any **red flags** for malignancy (unexplained weight loss, rectal bleeding, family history of bowel/ovarian cancer, change in bowel habit if aged more than 60). Other associated symptoms of IBS can include symptoms getting worse on eating, passing of mucus, lethargy, nausea, backache and bladder symptoms.

She is worried about her symptoms and wants to know the cause(s). Establishing her **health beliefs and ideas** about cancer are key. How did she form these? What has she read about ovarian cancer? She is right to be worried, as bloating was a symptom her mother had and this needs to be discussed again when incorporating her health beliefs in formulating a management plan.

Appropriate investigations to exclude other diagnoses recommended by NICE (1) are full blood count (FBC), erythrocyte sedimentation rate (ESR), C-reactive protein (CRP) and coeliac autoantibodies; CA 125 is not recommended as an investigation of bloating in a woman until aged 40 (2). Another test worth considering is the faecal calprotectin test, which is used to help distinguish between potentially serious inflammatory bowel disease (IBD) and less serious irritable bowel syndrome. In this case the rest of the history would be sufficient to help exclude IBD as a differential, so it would not be necessary. In this scenario it may not be essential to do all these tests on the first visit; an alternative could be a trial of medication and appropriate safety-netting to investigate if required.

Certain foods, dehydration and stress can precipitate IBS-type symptoms. These **possible triggers** need to be probed and alternative options given. For example you could say: 'You might want to consider cutting down on spicy food as it can trigger similar symptoms in some people. Other triggers could be caffeine, alcohol and fizzy drinks. We would advise a healthier diet with a good mix of vegetables and fruit.' If there is prominent wind or bloating, then limit fruit to three portions per day, including up to one portion of dried fruit if wanted. The recommended '5 a day' can be made up with vegetables. Potential stress as a trigger needs to be discussed sensitively, as this is not her primary reason for attending. One way to approach this might be to talk about exercise (walking, cycling or swimming) as a way of relaxing.

A **focused examination** would show that she is haemodynamically stable, she is not pale, she has a normal urine dipstick test and a negative pregnancy test. Check that there are no signs of an acute abdomen. A rectal examination would not be essential in this first consultation as many other features are pointing towards IBS as a diagnosis. However, if symptoms persist or if there is any rectal bleeding or ambiguity about the diagnosis, it would be good practice to offer this (with a chaperone).

Once you are confident of the diagnosis, **explaining** it in a way the patient can understand is very important. One way could be: 'You have a condition called irritable bowel syndrome, where the small muscles in the wall of your bowels contract and cause pain intermittently. Typically patients can get either looser or harder stools, with relief when you open your bowels, and sometimes worsening with certain foods or stress. Do you think anything might have triggered your symptoms recently?'

In terms of **management**, this patient really wants treatment to help her symptoms, so after lifestyle advice (for example, reducing fibre such as bran if loose stools, and increasing physical activity) discuss laxatives (avoid lactulose) for constipation, loperamide for diarrhoea, and consider antispasmodics such as buscopan or mebeverine for bowel spasms. Longer-term treatment such as tricyclics and selective serotonin reuptake inhibitors (SSRIs) would not be appropriate to start off in this situation, but can be considered later if required.

Appropriate **follow-up** (for example, 4 weeks with a symptom diary) and **safety-netting** are important. For example: 'I would expect your symptoms to improve with these simple lifestyle changes and medication; if they worsen or you develop any other symptoms such as loss of appetite or bleeding from the back passage, then please book a review sooner.'

References

1. National Institute for Health and Clinical Excellence (2008) *Irritable Bowel Syndrome in Adults: Diagnosis and Management of Irritable Bowel Syndrome in Primary Care.* London: NICE. http://www.nice.org.uk/cg061

2. National Institute for Health and Clinical Excellence (2011) *The Recognition and Initial Management of Ovarian Cancer.* London: NICE. http://www.nice.org.uk/cg061

Further Reading

British Dietetic Association and National Institute of Health and Clinical Excellence. Irritable Bowel Syndrome and Diet (patient information leaflet). http://www.nhs.uk/conditions/incontinence-owel/documents/nice%20guidelines%20ibs.pdf

PATIENT

Name: Ms Amber Smith
Age: 30
SH: Single mother, lives in a flat
PMH: Irritation of lateral cutaneous nerve of thigh. The patient is 3 months postpartum
DH: Nil of note

B2 Lower back pain (post-delivery)

Patient brief: Ms Amber Smith

You are a 30-year-old journalist who has a 3-month history of lower back pain. This started after the delivery of your first child. Your pain score, at its worst, is 5 out of 10.

Your pregnancy was uncomplicated, apart from requiring a ventouse delivery. You believe the pain is related to the epidural you had in labour (you are anxious about this if asked, as you have read horror stories on the internet about back pain following epidurals). You did not want an epidural on your birth plan, but had to change your mind due to the severe pains of labour. You ask whether epidurals can cause back pain and also why the hospital doctors did not explain this to you.

You are a single mother (no family nearby) and you are bonding well with your baby, who had had a completely normal 8-week check. She is bottle-fed and growing well. She is at nursery at present, as you need time to do some writing.

You have no urinary or bowel symptoms. Your periods have resumed. You have some numbness on the lateral aspect of your thigh, although this was also present during pregnancy when you had no pain. You were told by an osteopath in the past that this was lateral cutaneous nerve irritation of the thigh due to being overweight. You have not taken any painkillers.

Patient's opening remarks: '*I've just come in because I keep getting this sort of bad back pain down here…*'

Patient's agenda: You would like to know what's causing the pain, whether it's related to your epidural or something else, and some advice on what you can do for the pain. You would want a clear explanation of what physiotherapy can do for you before agreeing on this as a management plan.

Reflection

Key points

- **Data gathering:** Exclude red flags such as trauma/fall, urinary/bowel symptoms, new onset neurological symptoms. Appropriate focused back examination.
- **Management:** Check BMI with opportunistic health promotion around diet and exercise. Evidence-based approach to diagnosis and management of mechanical back pain.
- **Interpersonal skills:** Explore her health beliefs about epidural causing her back pain. You may need to address her question about why hospital doctors didn't explain this properly.

Suggested marking criteria

	Clear Pass	Pass	Fail	Clear Fail
Data gathering	Addresses differentials of back pain; social history reviewed, including bonding with baby and resumption of work	Social history reviewed; limited discussion around differentials	No exclusion of red flag differentials; limited social history established	No exclusion of red flags; no social history or discussion around diagnosis or management
Management	Correct examination and clear discussion of management options	Physiotherapy discussed with majority of advice	Physiotherapy or medication given without advice or follow-up	No advice, physiotherapy or medication given
Interpersonal skills	Establishes health beliefs, delivers information in bite-size chunks and summarises at the end	Establishes health beliefs and picks up cues; non-judgemental in consulting style	Fails to pick up cues, e.g. worries over epidural causing back pain	Didactic style of consulting with no emotion shown towards the patient

Trainer's comments

Back pain is a common condition in general practice, particularly in the ante-natal and postnatal periods.

This patient is 3 months postpartum, so a detailed **psychosocial review** is important during the course of this consultation. She is a single first-time mother with no family nearby. Is she coping well with her baby? Does she need any extra support? Are any friends available to help her? How does she feel now that her baby is at nursery and she is resuming work? Are there any issues with bonding with her baby? She may be fine with all of these issues, but it's impor-tant for you to explore them.

Exploring her **health beliefs** will reveal her ideas about the cause of her back pain. She has read about epidurals causing back pain and is anxious about this. What has she read? Who has she spoken to? What are her concerns in the short and long term? Did she feel pres-surised into having an epidural in the first place? Did she speak to her midwife and hospital doctors about this at the time?

Excluding **red flags** is important in both the history and examination (for example, PMH malignancy/HIV, bowels/urinary dysfunction, worsening neuro-logical symptoms, saddle anaesthesia, loss of weight, night sweats). Detailed questioning about her lateral thigh numb-ness will reveal that it was present before the epidural and her history of lateral cutaneous nerve irritation of the thigh has been given to the candidate.

The **examination** should include observation and palpation for any obvious deformities, checking range of movement and whether there is pain worsening on flexion, extension or both and checking lateral flexion. This should be followed by a lower limb neurological examination. Once your examination has excluded serious causes and confirms muscular pain, the skill in this consulta-tion is **explaining** this, taking into account the patient's prior health beliefs.

The association between epidurals and back pain is not clear. It is not thought to be directly causal, although prolonged lying in an awkward position rather than the procedure itself may be a factor. This level of discussion would be fine in this consultation, although you would be expected to **acknowledge the patient's concerns** that it was not discussed fully by the hospital team.

NICE guidelines on lower back pain discourage the use of lumbar spine X-rays and magnetic resonance imaging (MRI) for non-specific muscular back pain [8]. **Management advice** should include discussion on analgesia (par-acetamol first line and consider NSAIDs), encouraging **normal activities and staying physically active** as long as it doesn't make her pain much worse. It's important that you discuss this, given that her BMI is 33. You could also discuss postural advice when sitting (at her desk, for example) and safe lifting.

Physiotherapy could be a good management option if the patient is able to attend, as it would provide a thorough assessment and treatment for her muscular back pain. You should explain this clearly to the patient, as it takes time and requires commitment. An example would be: 'Physiotherapists can assess your pain in more detail and give you good advice on movement, posture and lifting. They can provide you with some stretching and strengthening exercises as well as manual treatment and even acupuncture. They can also recommend further investigations or referral if necessary. But physio does take commitment on your part to give it the best chance of working.'

Reference

1. National Institute for Health and Clinical Excellence (2009) *Early Management of Persistent Non-specific Low Back Pain*. London: NICE. http://www.nice.org.uk/cg88

Case B3

<table>
<tr><td colspan="2" align="center">**PATIENT**</td></tr>
<tr><td>**Name:** Mr David Jonsen</td></tr>
<tr><td>**Age:** 45</td></tr>
<tr><td>**SH:** Lives with wife and 5-year-old child</td></tr>
<tr><td>**PMH:** Nil of note</td></tr>
<tr><td>**DH:** No current medication</td></tr>
<tr><td>**Computer alert**: An alert pops up on your screen to remind you to ask about his smoking history and to check his blood pressure.</td></tr>
</table>

B3 Sexually transmitted disease (STD) and hypertension

Patient brief: Mr David Jonsen

You are a 45-year-old businessman and you don't come to the GP often. You are feeling embarrassed about coming to the GP with this problem: you have a clear, painless penile discharge.

You feel itchy but have not noticed a rash. You've just come back from a business trip to Thailand and had unprotected vaginal and oral sexual intercourse with an adult female you met there. You have not had any other recent sexual intercourse apart from with your wife (and you have always used a condom since).

You are worried about a sexually transmitted disease (STD), especially chlamydia. You know about it causing infertility. Your 35-year-old wife and 5-year-old child are regular attendees at this practice. You are worried about confidentiality and seek reassurance about this if the doctor brings it up.

You would like treatment for yourself and your wife. If asked, you will say you will tell her any medications prescribed for her are vitamin pills for '*health and energy*'. You would reluctantly agree to same-day attendance and treatment at an STD clinic but would prefer treatment by your GP. You agree to your BP check, but would only agree to follow up if you feel confident in your GP. You smoke 5 cigarettes a day.

Patient's opening remarks: '*It's a bit embarrassing, doctor. It's about my penis…*'

Patient's agenda: You are worried about an STD, especially chlamydia, and want treatment for you and your wife. But you don't want your wife to know that you have been unfaithful to her.

EXAMINATION FINDINGS

BP 145/94

Urinalysis: White cells + nil else

Genitalia examination: No rash, clear penile discharge, no offensive odour

Reflection

Key points

- **Data gathering:** Exclude red flags such as sexually transmitted diseases and urinary tract infection.
- **Management:** It's important to offer examination (with chaperone for intimate examination), evidence-based diagnosis and management of STDs. Consider referral to genitourinary medicine (GUM) clinic. Make the most of the health promotion opportunity: check BP and arrange appropriate follow-up. Discuss stress.
- **Interpersonal skills:** Explore his health beliefs about STDs, in particular chlamydia. Also explore any stress at home or work. While respecting patient autonomy and confidentiality, address the issue about treating the wife without her knowledge, clearly explaining that she has a right to know what she is taking.

Suggested marking criteria

	Clear Pass	Pass	Fail	Clear Fail
Data gathering	Discusses STDs sensitively; social history reviewed including strain on relationship	Social history reviewed; good discussion around STDs	Limited discussion around STDs; limited social history established	No social history or discussion around diagnosis or management
Management	Correct examination and clear discussion of management options, including referral to GUM clinic and BP follow-up	Medication prescribed with majority of advice but no referral to GUM clinic	Medication given without advice or follow-up	No advice or medication given
Interpersonal skills	Establishes health beliefs, delivers information in bite-size chunks and summarises at the end	Establishes health beliefs and picks up cues; non-judgemental in consulting style	Fails to pick up cues, e.g. worries over infertility and confidentiality	Didactic style of consulting with no emotion shown towards the patient

Trainer's comments

It is especially important to **establish rapport** in this consultation; here's a man who doesn't come to the GP very often and is presenting with an embarrassing problem. He may have more than one problem, and he may well only mention the penis discharge when he feels he can trust you. You need to use your **verbal and non-verbal communication skills** to make him feel at ease early on. Given the nature of the problem, and his worries about confidentiality about his infidelity, it is important for you to remain **non-judgemental** throughout.

You need to take a **detailed sexual history**. What are the symptoms (discharge/ rash/perianal problems/dysuria)? Was it an at-risk sexual contact (sex worker, sex abroad, intravenous drug use [IVDU]) and is she traceable? Male or female partner? Age of partner/any child protection issues? Use of condoms? Types of sexual contact (vaginal, oral, anal)? Last episode of sexual intercourse? Personal or partner's history of an STD?

This patient is aware of chlamydia, so **exploring his concerns** about this is relevant. Is he concerned about fertility as he and his wife are planning more children in the near future?

The key aspect of this consultation is how you address the **confidentiality** issue. This patient would need direct reassurances about this, as he is aware that his wife attends frequently. You should try to encourage him to discuss this situation with his wife, but if he refuses then your duty of care is first to him. It is important to talk about confidentiality and patient autonomy openly and confidently with him.

Although the exact nature of his STD is not yet identified, it would be reasonable (as long as he is using barrier contraception) to get him fully checked first at the **GUM clinic**; they could take urethral swabs for both cultures and sensitivity. The situation would be different if the partner in Thailand was under-age (you can break confidentiality in some specific child protection cases and you would also need to inform social services regarding his own child), or if he had an STD that would cause serious risk to the health of his wife (for example, HIV/hepatitis B/C) and he was not willing to use barrier protection or discuss the situation with her. The latter applies to serious communicable diseases, which the General Medical Council applies to diseases that can result in serious illness or death (1).

The discussion around giving her a '**vitamin pill**' to treat chlamydia should be dealt with firmly and confidently, again discussing confidentiality; remember, everyone has a right to know about their treatment. A patient who is not a healthcare worker may not appreciate the importance of these principles for doctors.

A referral to a GUM clinic would be the safest option in this situation, but GPs can of course also send swabs and treat as long as you organise appropriate follow-up. This would be an option if the patient is not keen to attend the local GUM clinic.

The patient's agenda will quite rightly be the focus of this consultation and take up the majority of the time. However, you have also been given instructions about an alert on the screen to check smoking and blood pressure. This is real-life general practice and you should address the **health promotion opportunities** if you can – even if it's simply a discussion with the patient about booking in to see your practice nurse to have a blood pressure check at a later date.

As this has been a complicated consultation and you have made an onward referral, it would be sensible to offer a **follow-up appointment** to discuss the outcome. This can also act to further develop the rapport you have built up during this consultation, especially as there may be important domestic issues looming for this patient.

Reference

1. General Medical Council (2009) Confidentiality: Disclosing information about serious communicable diseases. http://www.gmc-uk.org/Confidentiality_disclosing_info_serious_commun_diseases_2009.pdf_27493404.pdf

PATIENT

Name: Mr Nigel Dawes
Age: 30
SH: Lives in a flat, non-smoker
PMH: Nil of note, occasional hayfever
DH: Antihistamines

Last consultation: yesterday with another GP in the practice, for a repeat prescription for his antihistamines.

B4 Confidentiality and angry patient

Patient brief: Mr Nigel Dawes

You are a 30-year-old man and you are angry and upset because you saw the receptionist at this practice reading your notes as you left the building yesterday. You have come to complain about this to the GP. You know this receptionist as a 'busy-body' who lives in the same block of flats as you. You are certain that you are not mistaken; you clearly saw her reading your notes on her computer screen at reception.

You have never liked the way this receptionist has dealt with you in the past. She has been rude and never makes good eye contact when you speak to her. You've heard other people saying similar things about her.

You are not particularly stressed at home or work – you are just appalled at your confidentiality not being respected.

Patient's opening remarks: '*I'm sorry, but I want to make a complaint about your receptionist.*'

Patient's agenda: You have come to make a complaint about the receptionist breaking your confidentiality; you don't have any other medical agenda today. You want to know what the doctor and the practice are going to do about it. You want reassurances that this will be taken seriously and you would like to know the outcome of any meeting arranged.

If you are not happy with the doctor's manner, or their plans to address the problem, then you would like to know how to make a formal complaint.

EXAMINATION FINDINGS

Not applicable

Reflection

Key points

- **Data gathering:** It may be useful to explore his beliefs about why the receptionist would read his notes intently. Explore what has happened in the past.
- **Management:** It's important to offer a clear plan of action and to check whether he is happy with your suggestion. Discuss your complaints procedure and practice policy, including writing to the practice manager and response times. Offer a meeting with the practice manager and receptionist, or direct discussion by yourself. If necessary you could escalate the complaint to the health ombudsman or the clinical commissioning group (CCG).
- **Interpersonal skills:** It is very important to apologise appropriately to the patient early on for any distress caused (this is possible without apportioning blame if it is not yet clear where the blame lies). Demonstrating appropriate empathy may help to diffuse his anger. Show respect for his (and all your patients') confidentiality.

Suggested marking criteria

	Clear Pass	Pass	Fail	Clear Fail
Data gathering	Addresses patient's complaint sensitively and allows patient to tell the full reason; takes a social history to exclude other causes of stress	Addresses patient's complaint; limited discussion of social history	Doesn't fully address patient's complaint; no social history	Poor discussion about complaint with no social history
Management	Correct and clear explanation of the practice's complaints procedure	Correct discussion of complaints procedure	Limited discussion of complaints procedure	No discussion of complaints procedure
Interpersonal skills	Establishes beliefs, delivers information in bite-size chunks and summarises at the end	Establishes beliefs and picks up cues; non-judgemental in consulting style	Fails to pick up cues, e.g. worries over past behaviour of receptionist	Didactic style of consulting with no emotion shown towards the patient

Trainer's comments

Dealing with an angry patient is a difficult skill that requires **good communication** (see Chapter 6). It's important that he feels you have heard his story, so listen actively, showing authentic interest, and don't interrupt too soon. You need to make excellent eye contact and use paralanguage and open body language to encourage him to tell his story. **Apologising early on** for any perceived problems is usually a good start.

Finding out information from both sides is essential and you should make this plain with the patient from the outset. Why has this patient made this complaint *now*? Is he particularly upset with what he saw yesterday or has this been a build-up of small complaints against that receptionist? Have they had clashes in personality outside of the practice? The fact that the receptionist lives in the same block of flats is a sign that this needs to be explored further. This could be the main factor in this complaint, but you have not been able to discuss what happened from your receptionist's perspective as yet.

It may not be appropriate to bring up other possible stresses in his home or work life right now – it may sound as if you think he is over-reacting – but perhaps it's something to keep in mind for future consultations.

Apologising for any distress caused is appropriate, but you also need to spell out how you are going to deal with the situation. You need to show that you will take this situation **seriously** and look into finding out exactly what happened. You can disclose that you are unaware of any similar complaints made against this receptionist, but it's important to try to be objective about the situation and not come across as being defensive (or critical) without knowing the full facts.

In terms of **management**, you can mention that this is a **significant event** and detail how your practice deals with these: a minuted meeting of all team members to discuss the issue, what was done well and what could be improved. This would involve reflection on the whole event and suggestions for change – both for the individual and for the wider team – followed by a clear plan of action and follow-up to ensure it actually happens.

The significant event would cover the issue of **receptionists' access to patient notes**, where it is done and to what extent. For instance, can they access medical notes apart from basic demographics? What about blood results or clinician's notes? How much information are they allowed to access? This may vary greatly from practice to practice, but the general rule is that non-clinical staff should only have access to the minimum necessary clinical information.

GPs who are employers have to ensure that their staff are aware of standards of confidentiality. They should have systems in place to review, and if necessary audit, standards of **training** in patient confidentiality and the supervision provided for this. Perhaps the receptionists would benefit from refresher training in patient confidentiality?

Having explained this to the patient, he may still want to make a **formal complaint** and you should explain the process clearly in lay terms. Each practice should have a **complaints procedure** and the patient should be invited to write to the complaints manager (usually your practice manager), who can deal with the matter locally. The patient can also complain directly to the **commissioning body/ local CCG** instead. If local resolution is not possible, then the patient can refer the matter to the **Parliamentary and Health Service Ombudsman,** who is independent of the NHS and government. The patient can also access help and support in making his complaint from the **NHS Complaints Independent Advocacy Service**.

Further Reading

General Medical Council (2013) Treat patients and colleagues fairly and without discrimination. Good medical practice and duties of a doctor. http://www.gmc-uk.org/guidance/good_medical_practice/treat_fairly.asp

NHS Choice. Making a complaint: The NHS complaints procedure. http://www.nhs.uk/choiceintheNHS/Rightsandpledges/complaints/Pages/NHScomplaints.aspx

RCGP. Significant event audit. http://www.rcgp.org.uk/clinical-and-research/clinical-resources/clinical-audit/significant-event-audit.aspx

Case B5

PATIENT
Name: Mr Simon Tomson-Parker **Age:** 66 **SH:** Alcohol 6 units a week; smokes 10 cigarettes a day **PMH:** Gout, hayfever **DH:** No regular medication

B5 Hearing loss

Patient brief: Mr Simon Tomson-Parker

You are a 66-year-old former construction worker with worsening right-sided hearing loss for the past few months. Your wife is nagging you about having the TV on very loud and not listening to things she says. It is beginning to affect your mood (irritability, frustration, no sleep, appetite problems) and putting some strain on your relationship with your wife.

You enjoy a glass of wine about 3 times a week and you have not had any episodes of gout for the past 2 years. Apart from gout and hayfever, you have no other medical problems and for medication you only use a steroid nasal spray. You smoke 10 cigarettes a day. You drive a car and have not noted any problems with this.

You used to work in construction for 15 years and you are worried that the heavy machinery sounds you were exposed to could be causing your hearing loss. If questioned further about this, you used to drive machinery and were quite careful about wearing protective headsets, but are worried nonetheless. You are not in touch with any previous work colleagues to know if they have had similar problems.

You have not had any trauma, infections, fever, dizziness, balance problems, headaches or ear discharge recently. You have cleaned your ears with cotton buds every day for as long as you can remember, so if the doctor suggests that wax is the reason, you are dubious unless the doctor explains it properly.

Patient's opening remarks: '*I've been having problems with my hearing, doctor, and my wife's nagging me about it.*'

Patient's agenda: You want to know if there's a problem, what the cause is and what can be done about it, if anything. It's really starting to affect you and your relationship with your wife.

EXAMINATION FINDINGS

Weber's localizes to right.

Rinne's BC > AC on Right. AC > BC on Left.

Otoscope: Impacted wax + in right ear (unable to view tympanic membrane).

Reflection

Key points

- **Data gathering:** You need to exclude red flags such as trauma, vertigo, dizziness, balance problems, unilateral tinnitus (acoustic neuroma), infections (fever/vomiting/ear discharge/headache) or excess noise exposure.

- **Management:** Advise him to avoid cotton buds and use ear drops. Send for ear syringing only if problem continues after using wax softeners. Follow-up and review are important given the noise exposure risk factor.

- **Interpersonal skills:** Explore the patient's thoughts about the history of noise exposure and whether he wore protective headsets. Explore the relationship with his wife, irritability and mood, TV, exercises, smoking and alcohol (especially with regard to gout).

Suggested marking criteria

	Clear Pass	Pass	Fail	Clear Fail
Data gathering	Skilfully takes history of a hard-of-hearing patient. Puts symptoms in context of patient's social situation.	Exclusion or red flags; social history reviewed; appropriate examination	No social history established	No exclusion of red flags
Management	Explains diagnosis and management clearly; explains how to use drops and safety-nets	Medication with majority of advice	Medication without advice or follow-up	No advice or medication given
Interpersonal skills	Delivers information in bite-size chunks and summarises at the end	Establishes health beliefs and picks up cues; consults appropriately with a hard-of-hearing patient	Fails to pick up cues, e.g. worries over past exposure to heavy machinery sounds	Didactic style of consulting with no emotion shown towards the patient

Trainer's comments

A good candidate will adapt their **communication style** for the hard-of-hearing patient (see Chapter 6 for further discussion). That might mean speaking clearly, slowly at times, using non-verbal communication, active listening, bringing the chair closer to the patient and using writing material if appropriate.

Use open questions at the start to allow the patient to explain that his wife has encouraged him to attend. This should lead you to further exploration of the **psychosocial impact** of the condition. This will be the key aspect of the consultation. How is the hearing loss affecting him in his life? Is it having an effect on his relationship; if so, how long for? Has he noticed himself turning the volume up louder on the TV? Has it affected anything else, like hearing the telephone ringing, door alarms or wake-up alarms? Does he drive, and have there been any issues with this? Has it affected his mood – is he more irritable? Has there been any effect on his sleep or appetite? Has there been any impact on his balance?

It is important to take a detailed history to exclude any red flags or significant conditions that can cause **unilateral hearing loss**. Unilateral deafness, especially with tinnitus, vertigo or neurological symptoms or signs, should alert you to the possibility of **acoustic neuroma**. You should gather enough detail to differentiate between conductive and sensorineural causes. When did the hearing loss start? Was it a sudden or gradual onset? Is there also unilateral tinnitus? Has there been any obvious cause, such as excess noise exposure or trauma, or has he taken any ototoxic drugs? Is he systemically well; are there any infective signs or symptoms?

Exploring **health beliefs** may follow naturally from your noise exposure query or by direct questioning. Why does he feel that noise exposure from his previous job is having an impact now? Have any of his work colleagues been similarly affected or has he read anything about this?

The **examination** should include the correct use of a **tuning fork** and also an **otoscope**. The examiner will pay particular attention to how you **explain** what you want to do for the examination. An example for Weber's test could be: 'This is a tuning fork that I'm going to use to test your hearing… it won't cause you any pain. I'll just tap the ends to make them vibrate and place the other end on your forehead. Please tell me if you hear/feel it louder in your left or right ear, or down the middle.'

The **explanation of the diagnosis** taking into account the patient's health beliefs is another important skill that is tested in this station. Good candidates will incorporate the patient's own health beliefs into their explanation. The patient and the examiner will be looking for a clear explanation and checking that you avoid medical jargon.

Simple **management advice** would include avoiding the use of **cotton buds** (as this may push the wax in further and can cause abrasions in the ear canal) and encouraging the use of **ear drops** such as olive oil to soften the wax (either over the counter or prescribed). Most practices offer **ear syringing**, so you could discuss this as an option if things continue – but only after the use of wax softeners. Appropriate **follow-up and review** after 2–3 weeks would be reasonable, especially as there is a history of noise exposure as a risk factor.

Possible differential diagnoses for hearing loss:

Conductive hearing loss	Sensorineural hearing loss
Wax	Noise exposure
Otitis media	Degeneration (presbyacusis)
Otosclerosis	Trauma (fracture of petrous temporal bone)
Eustachian tube dysfunction	Tumours (acoustic neuroma)
Glue ear	Infection (e.g. congenital syphilis, meningitis)
Perforated tympanic membrane	Toxicity (aspirin)
	Ménière's disease
	Stroke
	Cholesteatoma

PATIENT

Name: Mr Graeme Sanders
Age: 46
SH: Lives in house with wife and son; smoker
PMH: Hypertension
DH: Amlodipine 10 mg (for the last 3 years)

Recent investigations
Last 3 BP readings: 138/83, 122/79 and 133/80
Recent fasting bloods (3 months ago):
HbA1c 6.1% (or 43.2 mmol/mol)
Fasting glucose: 7.2 mmol/l
Total cholesterol 5.0
Sodium 136
Potassium 4.6
Creatinine 80
Urea 3.8

B6 Erectile dysfunction and prescribing

Patient brief: Mr Graeme Sanders

You are a 46-year-old postman and you would like a prescription for Viagra (sildenafil). You are married with a 14-year-old son, but you have recently started an affair with an old school friend (female). You don't use condoms as she is on the pill.

You usually get normal erections, but that depends on the frequency of sex per week. You do not have diabetes, although It does run in the family (grandfather and uncle). You do not feel excessively thirsty, you are not passing urine more often during the day or night and you are not particularly tired. Your urinary stream is normal, you don't have to pass urine urgently and you don't have any discomfort passing urine.

You smoke 10 cigarettes a day and drink alcohol only on weekends. You have well-controlled blood pressure and have not had any side effects in the past. If the doctor tells you that you are not eligible for an NHS prescription for Viagra, then tell them that you are getting impotence as a side effect from your medication and that this has only started now (even though you have been on it for 3 years). You know about this from a friend as a way of trying to get free Viagra from your doctor. Your wife does not know about your affair and you have not had sex with her in more than 2 years. She is also a patient at this practice and you want assurances that the doctor will not tell her about your request.

Patient's opening remarks: *'This should be quick – I'm really here to ask if I can have a prescription for Viagra, doc.'*

Patient's agenda: You want a prescription for Viagra, preferably on the NHS, and you don't want your wife to know about it.

EXAMINATION FINDINGS

BP 122/78. P 70/min regular
Urinalysis: NAD
BMI 28
If asked, normal testicular exam

Reflection

Key points

- **Data gathering:** Don't forget to cover STIs, contraception, his raised HbA1c and diabetic control (repeat fasting glucose and HbA1c, dietary/exercise advice). Don't forget to cover cardiovascular risk factors, do an appropriate focused examination including BP, pulses and genitals, and consider checking testosterone and prostate-specific antigen (PSA) test after discussion.

- **Management:** Safe prescribing for erectile dysfunction (ED) and awareness of NHS indications. Discuss changing or cutting the dose of amlodipine. The ethical issues are to remain non-judgemental, respect patient autonomy and respect his confidentiality. Bear in mind the concept of justice and fair use of limited NHS resources.

- **Interpersonal skills:** The actor patient will be nervous and circumspect at the start. If you are non-judgemental and use good non-verbal communication, he will open up and talk about his affair. He will be confident with his request for Viagra. It's important to explore his beliefs about Viagra, its indications and usage. Ask too about the medication side effects he mentions. Don't forget about the relationship with his wife and how this may be affecting his son. What is his mood like at home and at work?

Suggested marking criteria

	Clear Pass	Pass	Fail	Clear Fail
Data gathering	Addresses raised HbA1c issue appropriately within context of consultation; social history reviewed, including strain on relationship	Social history reviewed; limited discussion around HbA1c issue	No social history established	No social history or discussion around bloods
Management	Explains NHS indications for ED medication clearly; arranges follow-up for repeat HbA1c	Medication prescribed with majority of advice	Medication given without advice or follow-up	No advice or medication given
Interpersonal skills	Delivers information in bite-size chunks and summarises at the end	Establishes health beliefs and picks up cues; non-judgemental in consulting style	Fails to pick up cues, e.g. worries over confidentiality of this consultation	Didactic style of consulting with no emotion shown towards the patient

Trainer's comments

This is a complex consultation that tests several different skills. **Non-judgemental communication** with this nervous patient will allow you to build rapport early on. Men do not visit their GPs regularly, so a consultation like this does represent an opportunity for **health promotion**.

This case tests your ability to **balance your agenda** (addressing the blood results and health promotion about diabetes) with the patient's agenda (getting help for erectile dysfunction). You need to manage this sensitively, especially given the psychosocial context. You should discuss confidentiality too, as his wife is also a patient at your practice. Are there any risks for serious STIs? How is his relationship with his wife and son? Are there any other stressors in his life, either work related or financial?

Although erectile dysfunction is not a life-threatening condition, it is closely associated with important physical conditions and can also affect psychosocial health. It is important to establish a **cardiovascular history** and to outline other risk factors (smoking, sedentary lifestyle, obesity, hypercholesterolaemia, relevant family history). This assessment of risk factors would provide you with an opportunity to discuss his blood results (borderline cholesterol, borderline raised HbA1c, raised fasting glucose) and to suggest further monitoring and thinking about health promotion. You might consider measuring free testosterone and PSA levels, after discussion with the patient.

Appropriate examination would include re-checking his blood pressure and pulses, checking his BMI and considering a genital examination. Digital rectal examination is not mandatory in every patient with ED, but you might consider it if there are genitourinary symptoms (1).

Starting an oral phosphodiesterase type-5 inhibitor (such as sildenafil) is appropriate as long as you have addressed potential causes and cardiovascular risk. The British National Formulary (BNF; 2) states clear indications for providing such medication on an NHS prescription – diabetes mellitus, multiple sclerosis, Parkinson's disease, polio, single gene neurological disease, prostate cancer, spina bifida, spinal cord injury, severe pelvic injury or surgery, dialysis, kidney transplant, and severe distress (only if assessed by specialist centres).

The usual frequency of prescription is one tablet per week. You should advise the patient to take one tablet one hour before planning to have sex. The tablet can be taken before or after food, but will take longer to work after eating a large meal. Most preparations should not be taken more frequently than once a day.

Side effects to mention include headaches, flushed face, indigestion and blocked nose. Occasionally blurred vision, dizziness and sensitivity of light can occur. If prolonged or painful erections lasting longer than four hours occur, then the patient should consult a doctor straightaway. Be aware that these drugs should be used with caution in people with cardiovascular disease and are contraindicated in patients taking nitrates, in whom vasodilatation or sexual activity is inadvisable, or in patients with a previous history of non-arteritic anterior ischaemic optic neuropathy (2).

The request for NHS rather than private prescribing of medication should be dealt with sensitively but firmly. As mentioned, there are clear criteria for this and you may be drawn into a discussion about fair rationing of NHS resources with some patients. Even if the patient does genuinely have impotence as a side effect of his medication, this wouldn't qualify him for private prescriptions – but you might consider a switch of his anti-hypertensive medication amlodipine to an alternative in case it was contributing to the problem. In this case, many candidates may go along with the advice of a confident patient who has said he has researched it on the internet, but for information a recent systematic review concluded that only thiazide diuretics and beta-blockers may adversely affect erectile function (3). ACE inhibitors, angiotensin receptor-blockers and calcium channel-blockers are reported to have no relevant effect on erectile function.

References

1. Hackett, G., Dean, J., Kell, P., Price, D., Ralph, D., Speakman, M. & Wylie, K. (2008) *Guidelines on the Management of Erectile Dysfunction*. Lichfield: British Society for Sexual Medicine. www.bssm.org.uk

2. British National Formulary (BNF). http://www.bnf.org/bnf/index.htm

3. Baumhäkel, M., Schlimmer, N., Kratz, M., Hackett, G., Jackson, G. & Böhm, M. (2011) Cardiovascular risk, drugs and erectile function – a systematic analysis. *International Journal of Clinical Practice*, 65 (3), 289–298.

Case B7

B7 Knee pain/weight loss/eating habits

Patient brief: Ms Karen London

You are a 20-year-old student who has recently started university; you have come to the doctor about your painful knees.

You are very conscious about being overweight and have started running recently. You are using an old pair of trainers from your flatmate, who has the same shoe size. You started running 2 months ago and are trying to run 3 times per week for about 15 minutes each run. You do this on the streets. You find that your knees are painful when running for more than 5 minutes. Your knees do not swell up, but they do click. You have pain that lasts for a few hours each evening. You have noticed pain on walking up stairs now and this has prompted you to come to see your GP. You don't have any morning or night pain or stiffness. There's no locking or giving way of your knee (if asked, you would like the doctor to explain what these terms are). You have not twisted your knee.

You know that your weight gain is due to polycystic ovaries, but you want to know if you will ever be able to do enough exercise to lose weight with this condition. If asked about your weight loss ideas, you admit to trying fad diets and are currently on a 'cereal diet' where two of your meals per day are Rice Krispies. You find that you binge in the third meal and snack on chocolates and crisps in between. You have never been sporty, but you're motivated by wanting to look thin for university. Your mood is fine, as are your sleep and concentration. Your periods are regular since being on the pill. You do not have acne or excess hair growth on your face.

Opening remarks: '*It's my knees – they're just really painful at the moment.*'

Patient's agenda: You want to know what's wrong with your knees, but you're also worried about your weight and would like some help and advice about weight loss.

Reflection

Key points

- **Data gathering:** Don't forget red flags: trauma (ligament/menisci damage) and infection (fever, hot swollen joint, reactive arthritis). Appropriate focused examination of the knee.

- **Management:** Give simple RICE advice (Rest, Ice, Compression, Elevation). Advise non-weight-bearing exercises like swimming or cycling, graded activities, NSAIDs and physiotherapy. Injections and/or surgical review are not necessary. Offer referral to the dietitian.

- **Interpersonal skills:** The actor will be anxious at the start. If you are non-judgemental and use good non-verbal communication, she will open up and talk about her knee problems in the context of her issues with trying to lose weight. Explore her health beliefs about knee pain and how she has been exercising. Try to address self-esteem issues, diet, appropriate exercise and mood. Adopt a non-judgemental, supportive approach to her weight problems.

Suggested marking criteria

	Clear Pass	Pass	Fail	Clear Fail
Data gathering	Addresses self-esteem issues appropriately within context of weight loss and increasing exercise	Exclusion of red flags, social history reviewed; limited discussion around diet	No exclusion of red flags or social history established	No social history or discussion of diet/exercise
Management	Simple RICE advice; non-weight-bearing exercises like swimming/cycling; graded activities; NSAIDs; physiotherapy; no to injections/surgical review; dietician referral or lifestyle review	Majority of advice; no referral to dietician	Medication given without advice or follow-up	No advice or medication given

	Clear Pass	Pass	Fail	Clear Fail
Interpersonal skills	Delivers information in bite-size chunks and summarises at the end	Establishes health beliefs and picks up cues; non-judgemental in consulting style	Fails to pick up cues, e.g. worries over weight loss	Directive or patronising with no empathy; allows personal views to offend patient

Trainer's comments

Although she opens with her knee pain, this young female patient has also come about her increasing weight, so will be understandably embarrassed or nervous. There may be complex underlying issues regarding her **eating behaviour** and you should gently explore this as the consultation proceeds. Good rapport and **effective communication** will help keep the patient at ease. The patient has taken the initiative to come in herself for this problem; what has triggered this?

She is trying to address her exercise, but her ideas about diet and eating need to be explored further. Fad diets should not be encouraged. We would advise a healthier diet with a good mix of vegetables and fruit, fish and white meat, along with good hydration. All may not be revealed about her eating habits in this first consultation, so an appropriate follow-up or referral to the dietician should be arranged. If there is a suspicion of an eating disorder, then ask about her mood, sleep and concentration. She has known polycystic ovaries, so you should also ask about her periods, acne and any hirsutism.

When you have established that her knee pain (and its relationship to her increase in exercise in order to lose weight) is her main complaint, then this should be your main focus. You need to ask some **focused questions** to make sense of her symptoms, perhaps **signposting** the shift in questioning style as you proceed. Is her pain always on weight-bearing exercises or does it occur after prolonged sitting as well? Was there any preceding trauma? Do stairs make it worse? Does she have many stairs at home, work or university? Is there any evidence of infection (fever/systemically unwell/hot swollen joint), underlying inflammation (morning stiffness, multiple small joint pain and swelling) or metastatic disease (night pain)?

The patient may ask for a **clear explanation** when asked about knee locking ('the joint getting stuck or blocked in a position making it necessary for you to manually unblock it') or giving way ('the joint buckles underneath you and feels unstable').

The **examination** should be focused and cover the main areas of any joint examination (observation, palpation, movement [active/passive/resisted] and special tests). Appropriate special tests for the knee would be checking collateral and cruciate ligaments (see Chapter 3).

Once you have established that there is no obvious structural damage, it's likely that her knee pain is the result of her increased weight gain. Now you need to **explain** the diagnosis clearly and go on to discuss what can be done.

You should **congratulate** her on starting exercising already. She should be advised to increase her **activity levels** gradually as the sudden change and increase in frequency and intensity of exercise will be contributing to her pain. In order to get on top of the pain she should rest the joint (relatively), apply ice (a wrapped frozen bag of peas on her knees for 15 minutes, 3 times per day), apply compression with a tubigrip bandage if there is any swelling, and elevate her leg when she is at home.

When her pain has improved she can first start any **non-weight-bearing exercises** such as swimming and cycling instead, as this will take the pressure off her knees. She can gradually increase her activities back to running, but in a graded fashion. She can get a short course of non-steroidal anti-inflammatory medication, either on prescription from you or over the counter, with the usual checks for any history of asthma or gastrointestinal problems. Referral to a physiotherapist for further review and advice would be appropriate, either at a follow-up appointment or in this appointment if the patient or doctor prefers.

A **follow-up** arranged in 2 or 3 weeks would allow you to monitor her symptoms and review her eating habits and activity levels.

Case B8

B8 Insomnia

Patient brief: Mr Sammy Patel

You are a 34-year-old man and you've been having trouble falling asleep for the past few months. You have come for some sleeping tablets.

You are in bed for 9 hours but you only sleep for about 6. You do not have any recurrent thoughts that keep you awake at night. You do not snore or wake up in the middle of the night gasping for breath.

You work as an odd-job man, but work is slow at present. You are single and live with flatmates. You drink 2 cans of strong beer 2–4 times a week and drink 3 cups of coffee per day. You smoke 15 cigarettes a day and have never taken any recreational drugs. You have never had any criminal convictions. You have financial worries, "as most people do these days".

You have started jogging in the evenings, but this has made things worse, if anything. You are irritable during the day and can get angry when you speak to your mother. Your appetite is OK and you eat a lot of fast food: pizzas, curries and burgers. You've always been slim; there's been no recent weight gain or loss.

You have never had counselling or been on antidepressants in the past. You have no thoughts of harm to yourself or others.

Patient's opening remarks: '*I'm having real trouble sleeping and it's getting desperate now. I really just need some sleeping tablets or something to help me sleep.*'

Patient's agenda: You want sleeping tablets, as you are getting very frustrated by your continual lack of sleep. You've tried over-the-counter products, which are 'useless'. You won't be happy unless you are given at least a short course of sleeping tablets. You have not felt like this before and are concerned that this will last for ever.

Reflection

Key points

- **Data gathering:** Cover red flags of alcohol/substance misuse, depression and anxiety. Make sure that you are clear on lifestyle details, especially coffee and alcohol and his fast-food diet.
- **Management:** Advise him to reduce coffee and alcohol and improve sleep hygiene (for example, discuss routine, avoid late exercise). Discuss benzodiazepines for short-term use only, and clarify long-term risks of dependence, tolerance, hangover. Consider a sleep diary.
- **Interpersonal skills:** The actor will be tired and irritable from the start. If you are non-judgemental and use good non-verbal communication, he will treat you with respect during the consultation. Explore health beliefs around insomnia, value of medication and links to exercise.

Suggested marking criteria

	Clear Pass	Pass	Fail	Clear Fail
Data gathering	Addresses insomnia and identifies causes (financial worries, alcohol, coffee, evening exercise); addresses mood, screens for anxiety/depression	Excludes anxiety/depression; limited discussion around diet/exercise	No discussion around alcohol/mood	No social history or discussion around alcohol/mood
Management	Simple advice re diet/exercise/sleep hygiene; skilfully deals with sleeping tablet requests and negotiates appropriately	Majority of advice; less negotiation	Medication given without advice or follow-up	No advice or medication given
Interpersonal skills	Delivers information in bite-size chunks and summarises at the end	Establishes health beliefs and picks up cues; non-judgemental in consulting style	Fails to pick up cues, e.g. financial worries	Didactic style of consulting with no emotion shown towards the patient

Trainer's comments

This patient is having trouble sleeping; he's likely to seem tired and be irritable from the outset. Poor sleep is associated with reduced physical and mental (depression/anxiety/alcohol/substance misuse) health. A **detailed history** should reveal any **depression or anxiety-related** issues. In this case there are no obvious triggers apart from financial worries, but this patient is unlikely to feel that these are contributing to his persistent insomnia. Talking in detail about his **caffeine and alcohol** intake is important, as is a detailed review of his **sleep routine**. Does he have a regular sleeping environment (the same bed, bedding, furniture in the bedroom and so on)? Is there any noise from flatmates that might be contributing? Does he exercise in the evenings or use a computer screen or watch TV in his bedroom at night?

Check for risk factors for obstructive sleep apnoea: obesity (especially large neck circumference), chronic snoring, gasping and breath holding, and daytime sleepiness.

If you haven't found an obvious cause for his insomnia during the consultation, then consider further **investigations** and think about your **management options**. You might consider the following tests, although in the absence of any specific symptoms or signs, they usually won't be required in the first consultation: FBC (anaemia), ferritin (low in restless legs syndrome), thyroid (hyperthyroidism), ESR (screen for inflammatory conditions).

The patient is keen on **sleeping tablets**, so you need to have a frank discussion about their short-term use and addictive potential (1). The doctor should also inform the patient of the benefits of non-drug-based treatments first. The patient should be encouraged to keep a sleep diary.

You'll need to discuss general **sleep hygiene**, even if the patient feels that his routine is perfect. The key points are: limit caffeine to one cup of coffee in the morning, avoid daytime napping, don't go to bed until drowsiness sets in, avoid late-night screens (for example, TV or computer), avoid regular checking of clocks, and regular exercise is good but avoid exercise close to the sleep period. If the patient is not asleep within 15–20 minutes, then he should get out of bed and return only when he feels drowsy.

The patient may well have tried over-the-counter **sleeping medication**, anything from herbal medication to antihistamines. He is therefore requesting hypnotic drugs (benzodiazepines or 'Z' drugs), which should only be prescribed for short-term use as they can cause tolerance, dependence and withdrawal symptoms. There is also the risk of misuse as they have a high 'street value', risk of overdose and potential effect on driving (1).

You should arrange a clear plan of action, with a **sleep diary**, and **follow-up** should be arranged with medication negotiated between the doctor and patient. This requires good communication skills throughout a potentially difficult consultation.

Reference

1. Falloon, K., Arroll, B., Elley, C.R. & Fernando, A. (2011) Clinical review: The assessment and management of insomnia in primary care. *British Medical Journal*, 342, D2899.

PATIENT

Name: Mr David Marron
Age: 36
SH: Nil of note
PMH: Anxiety
DH: No current medication

B9 Paternity testing

Patient brief: Mr David Marron

You are a 36-year-old carpenter and you would like to have a paternity test.

You have been suspicious for years that your 3-year-old son does not look like you, and you worry that your wife may have cheated on you years ago. In addition, some of your work colleagues have been winding you up about it, as your son has green eyes and neither you or your wife does (you both have brown eyes).

You, your wife and your son are all registered at the practice and you're all healthy and well. The purpose of the visit is to ask your GP to do a paternity test. You've looked on the internet and know that the test is non-invasive (just a swab in the mouth). You are happy to pay the fee required. You will bring your son in alone and under no circumstances do you want your wife to know. You do not want your GP to make a direct record of this consultation in your notes, as your wife knows one of the nurses (your children go to nursery together), but will agree if the doctor explains to you the nature of confidentiality.

You have felt more anxious recently as a result of this, but you are sleeping, eating and concentrating OK and your work as a carpenter is fine. You do not want any medication or counselling for your anxiety, as you feel that knowing the paternity test results will cure your anxiety. You do not drink excessively and have never taken any drugs. Your son is happy at nursery and you think it will also be in his best interests to know the results. You are not sure what you would do if you found out you are not the father, but you will take each step at a time.

Patient's opening remarks: '*Yes, I've come to talk to you about getting one of those paternity tests for me and my son. I've seen them on the internet – just a swab in the mouth, I think,*'

Patient's agenda: You want a paternity test; you don't want your wife to find out about it. You think that knowing the results – whatever they are – will help your anxiety.

Reflection

Key points

- **Data gathering:** You need to establish details of the relationships and explore the possibility of anxiety, depression and substance misuse. Consider any child protection issues.

- **Management:** It will help to have a sound approach to the ethical issues here: you need to balance the patient's autonomy with his wife's, while acting in the best interests of the child. You need to demonstrate respect for confidentiality, including of the patient, his wife and his son; it applies to all members of the practice. Discuss the implications of the test results beforehand, as this is potentially distressing information. Try to persuade the patient to discuss the testing with the mother; the BMA advises not getting involved without the mother's consent (1).

- **Interpersonal skills:** The actor will be anxious throughout the consultation. He is clear about his request and has researched it on the internet. Find out what he knows about paternity testing.

Suggested marking criteria

	Clear Pass	Pass	Fail	Clear Fail
Data gathering	Addresses paternity test request appropriately; social history reviewed including strain on relationship and work	Social history reviewed; limited discussion around paternity test request and its impact on the patient and his family	No social history established	No social history or discussion around reasons for request
Management	Explains how we can help and encourages mother to be included in discussion; does not get involved in 'motherless testing'; arranges follow-up discussion	Issues discussed and says no to motherless testing with majority of advice	Agrees to testing without advice or follow-up	No advice given
Interpersonal skills	Delivers information in bite-size chunks and summarises at the end; establishes health beliefs and appreciates complex ethics of the request	Establishes health beliefs and picks up cues; non-judgemental in consulting style	Fails to pick up cues, e.g. worries over confidentiality of this consultation	Didactic style of consulting with no emotion shown towards the patient

This case throws up some complex ethical issues. The key to this consultation is not your knowledge of the BMA guidelines on paternity testing (1), but how you communicate issues around confidentiality with this patient. If you are unsure about the detailed guidance, it's OK to say so and to offer to find out. The crucial aspect here is appreciating and addressing the ethical issues.

Summary of BMA guidelines on paternity testing (1)

It is now possible to use home testing kits (using hair follicle or saliva samples), which are available on the internet and sent off for analysis. Although you always need samples from both father and child, modern technology means that these days you don't actually need a sample from the mother in order to get a meaningful result. This raises the possibility of samples being tested without all parties knowing about it – but the BMA advises that we should not be involved in 'motherless testing'.

The law is clear that informed consent is required before a sample is taken, but people with parental responsibility can give consent on behalf of a child (2). As doctors, we should only get involved if we judge the testing to be in the best interests of the child. If a parent refuses to consent for paternity testing, then a court can issue a direction for the test to be carried out. That doesn't mean that a blood sample can be forcibly taken from them, but 'inferences can be drawn' about the refusal to provide a sample. Courts take the view that in the majority of cases the child's best interests are served by learning the truth.

The BMA guidance would prefer to see a requirement for all parties to give consent before paternity testing, but in the absence of such a legal requirement, the BMA advises doctors to 'encourage those seeking testing to discuss their plans with the child's mother and the BMA advises doctors not to become involved if that advice is rejected. Irrespective of the outcome, confidentiality must be respected and no information about the discussion should be passed to the mother or the child without the man's consent.'

Your key ethical obligations here are to act in the best interests of the child, and to respect the confidentiality of the putative father and the mother, both of whom are your patients. You should discuss the implications of the test results – they could be distressing and have life-long repercussions. It would be advisable to try to persuade the patient to discuss the paternity testing with the mother before going ahead.

You will need to gather information about the **patient's relationship** to the child and to the mother, and explore his **mood** – including his previous history of anxiety. The actor will be anxious through the consultation. He is clear about his request and has researched it on the internet. It's worth finding out **what he knows** about paternity testing: What has he read and who has he spoken to? What is his understanding of the significance in change in eye colour? Why is the paternity test so important to his relationship with his wife and son? Has he ever approached his wife about it? What would happen if he did?

With this information, you should be in a better position to **explain what paternity testing involves** in terms that are relevant to the patient, and to discuss the **implications of the results** for him and for his wife and child. You can make clear your duty of confidentiality, but explain that the current advice for doctors is not to get involved without the **consent of the mother**. It's worth trying to encourage him to discuss this with her, and let him know that you are willing to help in those circumstances.

References

1. BMA (2009) Paternity testing: Guidance from the BMA Medical Ethics Department. http://bma.org.uk/practical-support-at-work/ethics/ethics-a-to-z
2. British Medical Association (2009) *Human Tissue Legislation – Guidance from the BMA's Medical Ethics Department*. London: BMA.

Further Reading

Department of Health (2001) *Code of Practice and Guidance on Genetic Paternity Testing Services*. London: Department of Health.

Case B10

B10 Multiple sclerosis

Patient brief: Ms Sonia Marsh

You are a 38-year-old management consultant. You attended the optician with blurred vision a few days ago. She mentioned you had optic neuritis and said to come and see your GP to discuss further. She said she would send the GP the details. You weren't clear about the diagnosis, but you looked up optic neuritis on the internet; you turned off as soon as you saw multiple sclerosis (MS) being mentioned. You know that multiple sclerosis is an incurable disease of old age and have read that people can end up in a wheelchair.

You want to know more and how you could have caught MS. How will it be diagnosed? Your blurred vision has now got better, but you want to know what needs to be done now. You do not wear glasses. You're more worried about potential future implications than your vision.

Your mood is fine (before all this happened), you can occasionally feel tired, but your concentration and memory at home and work are fine. You are a single parent, not in a relationship at present, and you have an 11-year-old daughter. You want to know the chances of her catching this illness.

You have suffered from UTIs in the past (3 times, treated with 3-day courses of antibiotics), but you have always had control of your urine and bowel movements. If asked about numbness or tingling or muscular conditions elsewhere, mention that you had carpal tunnel syndrome during and after pregnancy and that the symptoms do still sometimes come and go (right thumb and forefinger numbness and tingling, although no symptoms at present). You do not smoke or drink.

You are physically very active and have recently started doing triathlons – you are also worried about this.

Patient's opening remarks: *"My optician said I should come and see you about this optic neuritis… I'm really worried about it…'*

Patient's agenda: You are very concerned about the possibility of multiple sclerosis, how you caught it, and the implications for you and your daughter. If the doctor suggests referral to a specialist, you want to know which type of specialist, how quickly you can be seen and what they are likely to do.

EXAMINATION FINDINGS

Normal visual acuity

Urinalysis: NAD

Normal wrist examination for carpal tunnel syndrome (*do not let candidate examine*)

Reflection

Key points

- **Data gathering:** Establish that there are no red flags (current/past visual symptoms, bowel/urine function and any musculoskeletal symptoms/peripheral neurological weakness). Explore psychosocial impact and worries about her family. Focused neurological examination.

- **Management** Consider appropriate referral to neurologist (and ophthalmologist), discussing stress and impact on various aspects in her life. Acknowledge no cure for this relapsing/remitting condition, but impart knowledge that its effects are variable, with some more serious than others.

- **Interpersonal skills:** A stressed but confident woman who is worried about her potential diagnosis of multiple sclerosis (MS). She is a good historian and so would respond to questions around ideas, concerns and expectations. She would like more explanation about the condition, its progression and management.

Suggested marking criteria

	Clear Pass	Pass	Fail	Clear Fail
Data gathering	Addresses patient's concerns re MS; detailed questions regarding visual, urinary and neurological symptoms; social history reviewed, including impact on work, implications for daughter and her exercise	Discussion of associated symptoms; discussion around management/ prognosis; social history reviewed	Limited discussion around associated symptoms of MS; limited social history established but not put in context of disease; limited discussion around diagnosis/ management	No discussion of associated symptoms of MS; limited history established; discussion around diagnosis or management
Management	Correct and clear discussion of MS; need for neurology referral and formal diagnosis and potential impact on life	Referral with majority of advice	Referral with minimal advice; not addressing impact on life	Referred to ophthalmologist
Interpersonal skills	Establishes health beliefs re MS; delivers information in bite-size chunks and summarises at the end	Establishes health beliefs and picks up cues; non-judgemental in consulting style	Fails to pick up cues, e.g. worries over work, daughter, exercise	Didactic style of consulting with no emotion shown towards the patient

Trainer's comments

This is a difficult case, as it involves breaking bad news (see Chapter 6) and **managing the concerns** and expectations of an anxious woman who has some knowledge about a relatively uncommon condition. This reflects real-life general practice where we are faced with patients who may have read about their symptoms on the internet.

The candidate already has some knowledge about her problems, but you should use **open questions** to gauge her understanding more fully. Maintain a **non-judgemental** attitude – don't criticise her ignorance, but help her to understand. What has she read about MS? Is the diagnosis confirmed on the basis of the optician's report? Acute, sometimes painful, reduction or loss of vision in one eye, optic neuritis, is a relatively common presenting symptom of MS – and anyone with a decline in visual acuity should be **seen by an ophthalmologist**. If no obvious cause can be found, the ophthalmologist may refer to a neurologist with MS in mind (1). She is particularly concerned about risk of transmission to her daughter, so her ideas of what MS is need to be explored. Further associated questions about any visual, bowel, neurological or musculoskeletal symptoms will be useful, although a full **formal examination** of any of these symptoms is not usually necessary at this first visit. In practice, clinicians may opt to do a quick neurological assessment at the first visit, but this should not delay any subsequent referral.

As a general rule, you should inform the patient of the **potential diagnosis of MS** as soon as a diagnosis is considered reasonably likely (unless there are overwhelming patient-centred reasons for not doing so). You should do this before undertaking further investigations to confirm or refute the diagnosis (1).

A **simple explanation** should use as little jargon as possible and incorporate what you already know about her understanding so far. MS starts in early adult life and is an **inflammatory disease** of the brain and spinal cord caused by a person's own immune system. It is **not an infection**, but inflamed areas become scarred within the brain or spinal cord. Bowels, urine, muscles and nerves can be temporarily affected, causing relapses. There are different forms and for many people with MS the disease causes little trouble. However, for others it leads to problems that can affect all aspects of their own life and that of their family.

It is important to get a quick diagnosis, so **referral to neurology** is the correct step. The diagnosis is clinical, but is aided by an MRI scan and visual evoked potential studies. **Management** is usually initiated in secondary care (for example, steroids, linoleic acid, assess motor and cognitive function at home, advice on work and exercise).

You don't need to discuss further treatment at this early stage, but it includes specific neurological rehabilitation if the disease progresses, aiming to limit infections and stress. At a later stage management may have to address worsening visual symptoms, fatigue, bladder control, sexual function, declining mobility, sensory and cognitive loss, emotional lability, depression, anxiety, speech and swallowing difficulties, spasticity, contractures and ataxia. The patient may know aspects of this, but this case does not require such in-depth knowledge about management of the condition. **Listening, being empathetic, explaining the condition and referring appropriately** should be the main emphasis in this case.

Reference

1. National Institute for Health and Clinical Excellence (2003) *Management of Multiple Sclerosis in Primary and Secondary Care*. London: NICE. http://guidance.nice.org.uk/CG8

Case B11

PATIENT

Setting: Telephone consultation
Parent: Mrs Rachael Mortimer
Age: 34
Occupation: Businesswoman
Child: Oliver
Age: 6
PMH: URTIs; nil else
DH: Nil

B11 Nocturnal enuresis (telephone consultation)

Patient brief: Mrs Rachael Mortimer

You are a 34-year-old businesswoman and you are worried that your 6-year-old son (he will be 7 in 2 months' time) is still bedwetting.

He does this about 4 times a week. It's an ongoing problem and he's never been dry. He doesn't soil his clothes at night; the problem is only with his urine. It's a fairly large amount, it happens in the middle of the night and he doesn't wake up. He has slept in his own room since the age of 6 months.

You once read not to blame children about bedwetting so you don't speak about it at all at home, including with your husband or nanny, hoping that your son would 'grow out of it'. Now that he hasn't, you're not sure how long to wait and whether he has a 'real' problem or not. It's a bit embarrassing, but you've been dealing with it by using bed protection and disposable night-time clothes (including elasticated nappies/pull-ups at night).

Your husband (who works with you in a very successful design business) doesn't want anything to do with the issue and you're now finding it difficult to clean Oliver and the bed sheets, particularly at weekends. You love your son and have a very good nanny to look after him during the week and occasionally at weekends. This nanny started 6 months ago and he prefers her to any other he's had previously.

You've tried giving him an expensive present each time he stays dry, but that hasn't worked. You admit you weren't very systematic about this, but you are a very busy person.

Oliver is a quiet child, but is growing and developing normally. He isn't 'rough and tumble' like you were as a child and he does pick up frequent coughs and colds. You've seen out-of-hours doctors about these colds on two occasions and the examination was normal apart from viral upper respiratory tract infections. You don't really discuss school in great detail with him, but his nanny says he does enjoy it.

Your mother-in-law said your husband was 'quite late by the time he was dry', but you're not sure which age and daren't ask him.

Oliver has never had a urinary tract infection and doesn't drink excessively nor had any weight loss. There is no personal or family history of diabetes.

You would agree to come in only if the reasons are properly explained, as you would prefer not to due to work commitments.

Patient's opening remarks: '*I wanted some advice about my son, who is wetting the bed most nights now and he is nearly 7 years old.*'

Patient's agenda: You want to know if there are any medications that he can take to prevent this. You want to know if it's normal or not. You are a bit embarrassed about it, and too busy really to come in to the doctor's to discuss it.

EXAMINATION FINDINGS

Not applicable

Reflection

Key points

- **Data gathering:** Establish that there are no red flags (daytime symptoms, infective symptoms, faecal incontinence, polyuria/polydipsia/loss of weight, developmental/growth problems, family history of diabetes/urinary problems, any potential abuse at home or school). Consider the psychosocial impact on her child and family life, and a busy/stressful environment. Check midstream specimen of urine (MSU) for infection and glucose.

- **Management:** This is about diagnosing and managing nocturnal enuresis. Assess whether she has enough time/support for conservative management. Discuss conservative management, fluid diaries, star charts. Negotiate appropriate follow-up, with the need to assess child and parents together (father also if possible). Mention the later option of medication if appropriate.

- **Interpersonal skills:** This is a busy woman who is not overly concerned but wants the problem sorted in the easiest way possible. She is a good historian over the phone and would like more explanation about the condition and its management.

Suggested marking criteria

	Clear Pass	**Pass**	**Fail**	Clear Fail
Data gathering	Addresses patient's concerns re incontinence; detailed questions regarding daytime symptoms, excluding infection, faecal incontinence and diabetes; social history reviewed, including impact on whole family	Discussion of associated symptoms and excluding diabetes; discussion around management/ prognosis; social history reviewed	Limited discussion around associated symptoms of incontinence; limited social history of family established, but not put in context of disease; limited discussion around diagnosis/ management	No discussion of associated symptoms of incontinence; no social history; inadequate discussion around diagnosis or management
Management	Correct and clear discussion of conservative management including fluid intake, use of alarms; supportive of child and family, 'no blame', arrange review with child and family together	Arranges review with majority of advice; addresses impact on family life	Referral to incontinence clinic with minimal advice and not arranging review; not addressing impact on family life	Referral to incontinence clinic
Interpersonal skills	Establishes health beliefs re incontinence, delivers information in bite-size chunks and summarises at the end	Establishes health beliefs and picks up cues; non-judgemental in consulting style	Fails to pick up cues, e.g. family worries, lack of dealing with problem	Didactic style of consulting with no emotion shown towards the patient

Trainer's comments

A consultation like this requires excellent communication skills, so there is additional difficulty as it is a telephone consultation (see Chapter 6). Since this mother is not known to you, it is important to **establish rapport** as best as you can and listen carefully for any cues.

She comes across as wanting the best for her child, but is not overly concerned.

Is that because she has read around the topic and spoken to friends or does it show a lack of insight? She and her husband have a busy life running a successful business – is this having an impact on her child's current condition and if so, is she willing to accept or deal with this? Of course, it is difficult to jump straight into issues like this at the start of the consultation, but **picking up on cues** as they come along might uncover some of her concerns.

You should also demonstrate awareness of **child protection** issues. This mother sounds caring, but it would still be important to find out if the child is happy and developing well, who else they spend time and bond with, and if there are any other concerns. Some of theses areas can be gently probed during the consultation, but one of the aims would be to establish enough trust for the mother to bring the child to see you for a **booked assessment**. If possible, it would be worth enquiring whether the father can also attend, as it highlights the impact on the whole family rather than only the child.

Bedwetting can have a profound impact on a child's behaviour, emotional wellbeing and social life. It is also very stressful for the parents or carers. Bedwetting more than two nights a week has a prevalence of 8% at 4.5 years and 1.5% at 9.5 years. Most expect to be dry by 5 years. The cause is often unknown and may be a combination of sleep arousal difficulties, polyuria and bladder dysfunction. Bedwetting also often runs in families, as seems to be the case here. **Excluding red flags with closed questions** is still important (and exclude a **urine infection** with an MSU – she could drop this in to the surgery). However, the real issue will be addressing the psychosocial impact of dealing with this on her child and family in a busy/stressful environment.

At this stage, before a face-to-face review, **treatment options** can still be discussed. This would include monitoring **fluid intake** especially in the evenings (but take care not to restrict diet apart from avoiding caffeine), and the **use of alarms** to wake the child so he can go to the toilet (not if infrequent, parents having emotional difficulties coping, or if showing anger to child). If alarms are used then continue until 2 weeks of continuous dry nights. Consider the use of a **reward or star system** for positive behaviour. This does not necessarily have to be only for dry nights – it can include stars for using the toilet before bedtime and helping to clean the sheets afterwards.

After a full review and trial of conservative measures, **medications** can also be used (for example, desmopressin), although they are usually reserved for children older than 7 years if conservative measures have failed. You should point the mother towards **community clinics or support groups** (such as ERIC, [1]), but it will still be important to organise a booked review with the child.

Reference

1. Education and Resources for Improving Childhood Continence (ERIC). http://www.eric.org.uk/

Further Reading

National Institute for Health and Clinical Excellence (2010) *Nocturnal Enuresis: The Management of Bedwetting in Children and Young People*. London: NICE. http://publications.nice.org.uk/nocturnal-enuresis-cg111

Case B12

B12 Pulmonary embolism post-Caesarean section (home visit)

Patient brief: Ms Maryam Hassan

You are a 38-year-old woman who has had an elective Caesarean section 7 days ago. You came home 2 days ago after an uneventful stay in hospital. They checked your blood tests on a number of occasions during pregnancy and in hospital and made small changes to your thyroxine dose without any problems.

Since yesterday you've been coughing persistently. You are concerned now as you're becoming short of breath, so you called your midwife who has arranged for the doctor to visit. You think it could be a chest infection. You couldn't come to the surgery as it's too difficult with the newborn and your 2-year-old son.

You have a sharp pain on your right lower chest wall on taking a big breath in. On direct questioning you have twice noticed some flecks of bright red blood while coughing. There is no calf swelling or pain, no fever or vomiting, no pain at your wound site and no vaginal bleeding.

You do not work and you live with your two children. You split up with your partner before your child was born and you don't really want to talk about that much as he's not in your life any more. There was a history of domestic violence if that issue is discussed. Your mother usually provides good support, but she is working at the moment. Your mood since your return home has been good.

Patient's opening remarks: *'Thanks for coming, doctor. I've got this terrible cough – do I need some antibiotics, do you think?'*

Patient's agenda: If the doctor mentions you need to go to hospital, you say you would prefer some painkillers or antibiotics, as you will have obvious difficulty with two young children. If you do go to hospital then your only option is to take the children with you. If this is the plan, then you request to go to the maternity unit.

EXAMINATION FINDINGS

Afebrile

Chest examination: respiratory rate 24, reduced right chest expansion, normal percussion normal breath sounds, pain on deep right inspiration

BP 114/80

HR 110 regular

Oxygen saturation 98% on air

Calf: Not red, hot, swollen or tender; no signs of DVT or infection

Abdomen: soft, non-tender, no signs of wound infection

Reflection

Key points

- **Data gathering:** Establish that there are no red flags (need to ask about chest pain, shortness of breath, fever, haemoptysis and calf swelling. Check if any abdominal pain or infection of wounds post-C-section). You could use the PE Wells Score to assess risk formally (1). Explore the psychosocial impact on her with her other child and her mother being at work. Assess her mood post-op and the level of support she has.

- **Management:** Explain PE as a likely diagnosis and the importance of hospital attendance and likely admission. The patient needs to understand why you feel it is important for her to attend now. Manage the situation with her children, call an ambulance and speak to the on-call obstetric (and perhaps medical) team to ensure she gets seen soon in hospital.

- **Interpersonal skills:** A home visit on a woman who is short of breath lying in bed. She is reluctant to go to hospital, so good communication skills will be required for her to understand the importance of attending today.

Suggested marking criteria

	Clear Pass	Pass	Fail	Clear Fail
Data gathering	Addresses patient's concerns re cough, shortness of breath, haemoptysis and pleuritic chest pain; appropriate questions around recent delivery and post-op progress; assesses social situation and assessing her mood	Makes correct diagnosis of PE and arranges hospital admission; social history reviewed	Limited social history established; limited discussion around potentially life-threatening condition	Missing PE as a diagnosis
Management	Correct and clear discussion of PE and need for emergency hospital admission; considers social situation and discusses with obstetric and medical teams	Refers to hospital with majority of advice; does not discuss with obstetric or medical team	Fails to send patient to hospital as an emergency	Manages the patient at home without adequate follow-up
Interpersonal skills	Establishes understanding regarding PE, delivers information in bite-size chunks and summarises at the end	Establishes health beliefs and picks up cues; non-judgemental in consulting style	Fails to pick up cues, e.g. worries over children and her reluctance to accept the urgency of hospital attendance	Does not explain a potentially life-threatening situation properly and allows the patient to stay at home; no emotion shown to the patient's situation

Trainer's comments

Pulmonary embolism is a potentially life-threatening condition and this patient has a number of risk factors, signs and symptoms that point towards the diagnosis. In this case clinical findings of tachypnoea, tachycardia and reduced right chest expansion would confirm the likely diagnosis even in the presence of normal oxygen saturations.

Her **health beliefs** are different – she is unsure what the cause could be, apart from maybe an infection, but she doesn't think it could be serious. Being asked to go to hospital for likely admission is not an option she had been considering, so it will come as a surprise for her and she could be resistant if you don't explain the reasons properly.

This is an example of a case where the **management plan** would have to be more **doctor-centred**; there is little room for sharing options here. However, the patient still needs to be treated with full respect and her potential condition needs to be fully explained with jargon-free language. Ultimately, if she has capacity then it is still her decision whether she goes to hospital or not. Your role is to make sure she fully understands why hospital attendance is necessary in order to make an informed decision to go.

Once she has agreed, if there are any factors that cause difficulty, such as her children in this case, it is important for the doctor to be flexible and think of sensible practical ideas to help overcome the difficulty. This is where options become a possibility and you can take a more **patient-centred approach**. Can someone else come and look after the children? What support does she have – she has mentioned her mother as her main source of support. And how much is her partner now involved – are there any risks or issues regarding domestic violence that need to be addressed?

For **hospital attendance**, how is transport going to be arranged? Is it an urgent blue-light ambulance or a non-urgent one within the next few hours? In this situation, the safest option is an **urgent ambulance** and you can offer to stay to help make some calls for her regarding her children while the ambulance arrives. Can the children go with her? Where is the best place for her to be – on a medical ward or a maternity unit? This is important to her and if she prefers to be on the maternity unit then offering to make phone calls to both teams would help reassure her that you are doing everything you can to help her.

Reference

1. Nice Clinical Knowledge Summaries. Pulmonary embolism (revised June 2013). http://cks.nice.org.uk/pulmonary-embolism

Case B13

B13 Allergic rhinitis

Patient brief: Mr Jacques Hayward

You are a 33-year-old salesman, troubled by recurrent sneezing and a runny and blocked nose. Occasionally you get runny eyes, but your nose symptoms are the worst. You've been to the doctor once before for this and had a rushed consultation, which ended up in the doctor prescribing antihistamine tablets that you could have bought cheaper directly from the chemist. You've tried every single antihistamine tablet from the chemist and none seems to work fully, even the drowsy ones.

Your symptoms affect both nostrils the same, there is only ever clear discharge, no fever, no rash, no change in smell, facial pain, cough, wheezing or shortness of breath. You have eczema and use plain moisturising cream for this. You had mild asthma as a child, but haven't used an inhaler for 20 years.

You currently take cetirizine tablets twice daily and piriton tablets three times daily, which take the edge off your symptoms.

You are fed up now as the problem is having an impact on your work (you work in sales in a clothes store) and on your general quality of life. Constantly sneezing in front of customers is embarrassing and you need to look clean and presentable at your place of work. It can affect your sleep at night unless you take your piriton tablets.

You've just moved in with your girlfriend and she has a pet dog (a greyhound called Bolt) who you take out for morning walks. He doesn't shed much hair, but he does sleep in the same room as you both. You're not sure if this is the cause, as your symptoms have never really been under control even before you moved in. The symptoms were never this bad before you came to London 4 years ago (from South Africa). There is no way your girlfriend would get rid of her dog, and you wouldn't want that either. You could try sleeping in another room if that comes up.

You have not changed any bed linen since you've been there or used any protective bedding (only mention this if the doctor asks). It's a carpeted house and, if this comes up, you would not be able to afford to change to wooden flooring.

You thought you would give seeing your doctor another chance, otherwise you'll start trying some homeopathic treatment that a friend has mentioned in passing. You don't know much about this, but 'anything is worth giving a go'.

You have never tried any nasal sprays and this time you would like a clear explanation if any are suggested. You prefer not to carry anything in your pockets, so you will only take the nasal sprays if the reasons are properly explained.

You would like to get referred to a specialist for allergy testing at this visit, but would agree to a trial of different medication and a follow-up review if the doctor explains this clearly and confidently.

Patient's opening remarks: *'I've got a constant blocked and runny nose and I'm sneezing all the time. It's getting ridiculous now – is there anything you can do for me, doctor?'*

Patient's agenda: You need the problem solved this time as you felt a bit let down at your last visit 9 months ago. The consultation felt rushed and you were prescribed something you could have bought more cheaply anyway. You don't want to complain about the last consultation but would like to get your problem sorted this time.

EXAMINATION FINDINGS

Afebrile

Allow the doctor to examine the nose: Normal (no swelling/polyps/deviated septum) no tenderness

If chest examination is offered then say it is normal.

Reflection

Key points

- **Data gathering:** Establish that there are no red flags (purulent discharge, fever, rash, change in smell, facial pain, cough, wheezing or shortness of breath). Establish whether there are any potential allergens and what treatment he has already tried. Examine the nose and take a temperature.
- **Management:** Continue antihistamine use, add an intranasal steroid spray, consider short-term decongestants, address potential allergens, negotiate with regard to allergy testing and arrange appropriate follow-up.
- **Interpersonal skills:** Establish why he has attended using open and closed questions appropriately. Listen to his story. Apologise appropriately for his experience at the last consultation and take his problem seriously.

Suggested marking criteria

	Clear Pass	Pass	Fail	Clear Fail
Data gathering	Addresses patient's concerns re allergic rhinitis and the impact it is having on him; detailed questions regarding symptoms; social history reviewed including impact on home and work life; focused examination	All red flags established, as well as social history	No allergen history, social history re housing, work; not asking about what treatment has been tried	No red flags asked about; no allergens asked about
Management	Discussion on medication, nasal sprays, allergens and addressing psychosocial impact; negotiating specialist referral	Discussion on antihistamines, nasal sprays, addressing potential allergens	Some advice on antihistamines, no trial of intranasal sprays, referral to specialist	No further advice on managing this condition away from referring to specialist
Interpersonal skills	Delivers information in bite-size chunks and summarises at the end	Picks up cues about work; safety-nets; shows empathy towards impact on work/home life	Fails to pick up cues, e.g. worries over work/potential allergens	Didactic style of consulting with no emotion shown towards the patient or their situation

Trainer's feedback

Allergic rhinitis is a common condition that should be easily diagnosed and managed effectively in general practice.

This is a reasonable but 'fed-up' man who now wants to get this problem solved. He wants **clear explanations** regarding what the problem is and how it is going to be treated. Addressing this and his poor experience in the past is important, but if he does not want to complain about the previous encounter it is reasonable not to push this too much. His aim is to get the problem sorted now and for the future.

Open questions from the start will allow him to tell his story and how the condition is affecting him. His frustration at the continuing symptoms should be evident. Further probing will allow exploration of his health beliefs and the **psychosocial impact**. Does he feel that exposure to the dog is the cause, or is it a change in weather or climate from South Africa? Is it solely the condition that's having an impact or is there any underlying stress? Is his partner supportive? Is she affected?

Asking directly about **allergens** is important as it may affect management. Consider house dust mites, grass, pollens, allergens carried on animal hair, and work-related allergens such as latex gloves and wood dust.

You would be expected to carry out a **simple examination** of the nasal passages, checking for swelling, polyps or a deviated septum. Check his temperature too.

You can suggest **allergen avoidance**, but this may be tricky in this situation as a pet is involved. There may be no room for discussion in this matter, but you could suggest trialling the pet sleeping in another room, followed by deep cleaning the room, washing all bedding at 60 °C and using protective bedding. Having wooden/hard floors is preferable but not always possible, as is the case here.

Allergy testing can be useful if the trigger is unclear from the history or if symptoms are persistent or poorly controlled. In this case **intranasal sprays** (steroids or decongestants) have never been tried, so a **trial and review** policy would be the preferred management plan if the patient agrees.

Intranasal corticosteroids are a good first-line treatment and generally have similar efficacy. Different preparations can be prescribed according to local policy and clinicians' preference. They can safely be used long term as low-dose ones tend not to have systemic absorption, something that you should explain to the patient.

Intranasal decongestants can be bought over the counter and work well in the short term (7 days). Long-term use can cause side effects, including rebound nasal congestion, and over-use can cause hypertrophy of the nasal mucosa and subsequent worsening of symptoms.

In this situation a trial of an intranasal spray, attempt at allergy avoidance and **follow-up** in 3–4 weeks with a **symptoms diary**, would be a sound management plan.

Further Reading

NICE Clinical Knowledge Summaries. Allergic rhinitis. http://cks.nice.org.uk/allergic-rhinitis#!topicsummary

World Organisation of Family Doctors (WONCA) (2007) Management of Allergic Rhinitis and Its Impact on Asthma. http://www.whiar.org/docs/ARIA_PG_08_View_WM.pdf

Cases (C)

How to Pass the CSA Exam, First Edition. Imtiaz Ahmad, Raj Nair, Martin Block and Graham Easton.
© 2015 John Wiley & Sons, Ltd. Published 2015 by John Wiley & Sons, Ltd.

Case C1

PATIENT

Name: Mr David Perez

Age: 27

SH: Smokes 20/day, occasional alcohol. Lives in a rented flat with partner and young son

PMH: Nil of note

DH: Takes paracetamol during headaches

C1 Headache

Patient brief: Mr David Perez

You are a 27-year-old waiter and you moved to the UK just over a year ago from Madrid, as you were unable to find work at home. You have been working in a busy restaurant for a year. You enjoy the social aspect of the job but you have been working long hours, especially over the last 3 months since the owner sacked one of the other waiters.

The days are hectic: most days you finish after midnight, and you keep going by drinking 10 or more cups of coffee during the day. Your diet is erratic: you grab a snack mid-afternoon and eat a 'ready meal', or warm up something your partner, Lucia, has cooked for you when you get home in the evening. It often takes a long time for you to get to sleep.

You have had occasional headaches before (usually once or twice a year) but have never discussed these with a doctor. The headaches tend to last throughout the day. Features are:

- throbbing
- tend to be more pronounced over the left side of the head
- accompanied by sensitivity to light and to sound
- no visual symptoms
- no fever/rash

When the headaches occur you feel best if you can go to a dark room and sleep.

Over the past six months they have been increasing in frequency and duration. Initially they happened once a month, but over the past 3 months you have been having headaches every 1–2 weeks. They are now lasting up to 3 days. Their severity is 8–9/10.

You take paracetamol on one or two days in a week. You have not experienced any weight loss or vomiting. The headache can occur at any time of the day and is not worse if you sneeze or cough. It tends to help to lie down in a dark room.

Sometimes you have tried to work with the headaches (but you feel terrible when you do) and sometimes you go 'off sick' with them (but you worry that your boss may fire you if this continues).

You are struggling financially. You are supporting your partner and your son.

One of your brother's friends had a brain tumour and you are worried that there may be something serious going on here. If you are given space within the consultation you will voice these concerns.

You recognise that your lifestyle may be contributing to the headaches, but you're not sure what you can do to change this. You would be very keen to try any kind of preventative measures that are offered to prevent these headaches.

Patient's opening remarks: '*I'm having constant headaches, doctor.*'

Patient's agenda: You are worried about the cause of the headaches and are concerned that there may be something serious going on. The headaches are having a significant effect on your life and you are keen to do anything to prevent them. You are worried you may lose your job.

EXAMINATION FINDINGS

BP 112/78
No focal neurological signs or temporal tenderness
Cranial nerves 2–12: normal, intact
Afebrile, no rash

Reflection
Key points
- **Data gathering:** Take a clear headache history, detailing the frequency, intensity, duration and associated features. Exploring triggers, patient's understanding and the impact of the condition on the patient's life are important. It is also important to exclude other common causes of headache (for example, medication overuse, tension) as well as serious causes.

- **Management:** This must begin with a clearly described positive diagnosis of migraine. The shared management plan should cover treatment of the acute attack, a discussion around triggers and a consideration of migraine prophylaxis.
- **Interpersonal skills:** Listen to the patient's story with sensitivity. Work collaboratively with the patient in consultation.

Suggested marking criteria

	Clear Pass	**Pass**	**Fail**	**Clear Fail**
Data gathering	Takes clear and comprehensive headache history and gains clear understanding of possible triggers	Takes clear headache history	No information gathered on impact of condition and patient's worries about losing job	Insufficient information gathered to exclude serious cause for headache
Management	Patient leaves the consultation having strong ownership of the plan	Covers treatment, prophylaxis and triggers with clarity	Plan focuses almost exclusively on treatment of acute attacks	No clearly explained positive diagnosis of migraine
Interpersonal skills	Uses reflective questioning to encourage patient to come up with solutions around triggers	Explores impact with sensitivity to patient's predicament	Fails to pick up cues, e.g. worries over serious cause of headache	Didactic style of consultation

Trainer's comments

When gathering the **headache history** it is important that the candidate covers:

- Quality of attacks (intensity, site, associated symptoms)
- Timing and frequency of attacks
- Possible triggers
- Relieving factors
- Exploration of different possible types of headache present (you need to exclude a medication over-use headache, for example)
- Exclusion of red flags (for example, thunderclap onset, headache waking from sleep, new neurological signs, becoming progressively more severe)

The patient has several possible triggers for migraine (stress, tiredness, erratic eating habits, caffeine); exploring these is an essential part of data gathering and will also help in forming a management plan.

Sometimes working with the patient to map the headache frequency and severity graphically will be useful in clarifying the picture, see Figure 7.1

Enquiring about the **impact** of the condition is vital and must be done with sensitivity – the patient is in a vulnerable position if he loses his job.

Time management is important here. A common mistake is to spend too long on the data-gathering side of the consultation (especially in cases like this, where there is quite a lot of data to gather) and to neglect aspects of the management plan (which also has much to include). It is important that you achieve a balance here. You need to cover the key areas

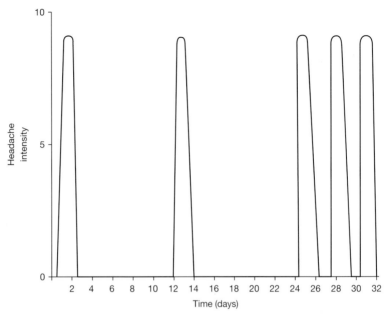

Figure 7.1 Showing an increase in headache frequency in a patient with migraine.

while listening to the patient and not making him feel rushed. A couple of ideas you may want to try to help with this are:

- **Do not interrupt the patient during the opening exchanges**. Allow him time to talk – the patient will often provide you with the crucial information.
- **Do not waste time repeating** the history. For example, if a patient has said early on that they are worried about a possible brain tumour (and you have responded to this cue with sensitive curiosity at the time), don't then waste time later asking 'Is there anything you are worried this might be?'

It is important that you spend enough time on management. Remember that this section should take up half of the consultation – there is a lot to cover here, including treatment of the acute attack, triggers and early discussions about prophylaxis. You should not overload the patient; break the information up as you go along, regularly bringing the patient into the discussion and allowing him to work with you to agree on a plan.

This part of the consultation should begin with a **clear positive diagnosis of migraine**. A patient information leaflet may be useful here. The best explanations are framed by the patient's understanding and context.

Discussion on treatment of the **acute attack** should cover prompt analgesia. Current NICE guidance is to offer combination therapy of an oral triptan plus NSAID or paracetamol [26]. Monotherapy can also be offered. Again, a patient information leaflet may be helpful.

There should also be a discussion on prevention of attacks, with the patient being encouraged to reflect on what he could do to decrease the risk of headaches. Additionally, the candidate should explore **prophylaxis** (for example, with propranolol).

A **headache diary** may be useful in giving the patient a clearer idea about triggers and may motivate him to undertake the necessary changes. This will also be useful when reviewing the patient at the follow-up appointment.

It would be good practice to arrange **follow-up** to review progress and response to treatment. The timing of this would depend on the agreed plan. If the patient has started prophylaxis this should be in 2–3 weeks; if focusing on triggers and a headache diary it could be longer (1–2 months).

Reference

1. National Institute for Health and Clinical Excellence (2012) *Diagnosis and Management of Headaches in Young People and Adults*. London: NICE. http://guidance.nice.org.uk/CG150

Further Reading

British Association for the Study of Headache (BASH). Guidelines for all healthcare professionals in the diagnosis and management of migraine, tension-type, cluster and medication-overuse headache. http://www.bash.org.uk/wp-content/uploads/2012/07/10102-BASH-Guidelines-update-2_v5-1-indd.pdf [NB: *These guidelines have been specifically mentioned in the examiner's feedback for the AKT exam*]

NICE Clinical Knowledge Summary. Headache assessment. http://cks.nice.org.uk/headache-assessment

Case C2

C2 Elder abuse (home visit)

Patient brief: Mr Alfred Barnes

You are an elderly retired bus driver. You are largely housebound due to a combination of joint pains, general physical frailty and a slight loss of confidence. You don't really get out much except for an occasional family get-together.

You have called the doctor out as you have had a nasty cough for the past week. This has worsened over the last 2 days and you are now coughing up thick green phlegm and having some intermittent fever. There is no shortness of breath, blood in sputum or chest pain.

If you are asked anything about your ideas, concerns or expectations about your cough you will reply that you '*just want something for the chest*'. You think you probably need some antibiotics.

When the doctor examines your chest, there is a large area of bruising on your back and a single bruise on the front of your chest. If the doctor asks more about this, you will at first go quiet and if the doctor asks sensitively you will talk further about the causes of the bruising.

The bruising has come about because your daughter, Jill, often gets angry with you. You blame yourself for this: '*I'm such a burden to her, she has to help me get dressed and everything*.' Last week she lost her patience with you and, during an argument in the bathroom, she pushed you hard and you fell heavily against the sink (hence the bruises on your back). She has hit you on four or five other occasions. She often refers to you as a 'silly old fool'. You will not mention anything about abuse unless the doctor comments about the bruising.

In spite of this abuse, your daughter buys you your paper every day (*Daily Mirror*), washes and dresses you and makes all your meals (which are delicious).

You suspect that Jill is not very happy. She is, in your words, '*always miserable*'.

You are scared of your daughter and if the doctor recommends telling social services you are very apprehensive about this. If the doctor mentions contacting the police, then you will say categorically '*No, this is not what I want at all*'. You feel vulnerable because without your daughter you don't know how you would cope. You will agree to adult social services referral if you feel confident in the doctor.

You have never been offered or considered home help.

If you feel you can talk to the doctor, you may divulge that you were quite a tough father when Jill was growing up and that you are worried she may be finally getting her own back.

Patient's opening remarks: '*Hello, doctor, I've got this terrible cough so I thought I'd better come and see you.*'

Patient's agenda: You think you need some antibiotics for a chest infection. You are apprehensive about getting into details about the abuse, but will do so if you feel you can trust the doctor.

EXAMINATION FINDINGS

Pulse: 88 regular. BP 138/84
Temp: 37.4
Resp rate: 14
Chest: crepitations right mid-zone

Information for candidate: Large 'bar-like' bruise across back, in a horizontal line, lower thoracic area. Smaller 4 cm round bruise at front of chest.

Reflection
Key points
- **Data gathering:** Don't waste too much time exploring ICE at the beginning; the real issues won't come out until you've seen the bruising. Explore the history of the abuse, its impact and the patient's thoughts on it.

- **Management:** While respecting autonomy, you must be mindful of risk to the patient – with appropriate involvement of social services.
- **Interpersonal skills:** You should engender trust through warmth, sensitivity and active listening.

Suggested marking criteria

	Clear Pass	Pass	Fail	Clear Fail
Data gathering	Explores at a deeper level the complexity of the relationship between Alfred and Jill	Sensitively elicits history and characteristics of abuse	Spends disproportionate time on chest infection (and associated ICE questions) without giving enough time to key priority in consultation – sensitive management of elder abuse	Does not uncover abuse/ neglect. Gives up too easily
Management	Alfred has ownership of plan and confidence in it	Involves adult protection team with Alfred's consent	Excessively didactic without seeking to engage Alfred in plan	Does not touch on key priority in the consultation
Interpersonal skills	Communicates warmth, empathy and respect	Gives patient space and encouragement to tell story and express fears	Does not fully explore psychosocial context	Does not show compassion to patient

Trainer's comments

This is a case of **elder abuse** and needs to be taken seriously.

The case will require some **flexibility**. If you waste too much time exploring an agenda that isn't apparent before the examination, then you will have less time to explore the real crux of this consultation – how to react to elder abuse in a man who is reluctant to accept help.

In the CSA, each case should have something to get your teeth into, some kind of specific challenge. This could be considered to be **the main priority** of the case. If the case seems too straightforward at first, keep an eye out for the **cues** that may lead you to where it's really going.

There is a lot to explore in your **data gathering**, including the history and features of abuse (physical and emotional). You also need to ask specifically about neglect and explore the patient's perspective on this (in this case, probably fear and reticence).

Throughout, you should adopt a style that engenders trust and respect. Use open and sensitive listening to encourage the patient's contribution. It may not be easy for Alfred to open up, so you'll need some gentle encouragement and some patience.

It is worth exploring the **social arrangements**. Does the daughter have a partner? Who else visits the home? Are there any other family members present?

What is the history of their relationship – did he ever beat her when he was younger (though this wouldn't excuse the current behaviour)?

Your data gathering should include an **assessment of the safety** of this man: is he in an immediate danger or not?

There is also the question of the **cough**, although it should not take you too long to gather the necessary specific data here. You will run into problems if you spend too long here or allocate an excessive amount of time to 'ICE' questions. However, it is important that you gain a clear idea of the symptoms and duration of this illness.

You will need to be very sensitive when it comes to **management**. There are some key points you will need to consider:

- Do you feel confident that the patient has the capacity to make a decision about his future? This would seem to be the case. You should respect Alfred's autonomy.
- What is the immediate risk?
  It would be sensible to involve the adult safeguarding team (which will be part of local social services), but how are you going to do this?

  Finally, it is important to bear in mind that if you deem the patient to be at significant risk of immediate harm and he does not want to take this further, this is

an instance where you should consider **breaking confidentiality** in speaking to the adult protection team. If this is something you are considering, then you should communicate this to your patient.

Other services you may want to consider involving in this case could include Age Concern, voluntary befriending services, district nurses and the local elderly day-care hospital.

You will have to balance the need for ongoing relationship building (which in this case will be grounded in sensitivity and respect for the patient) with your concerns for the patient's safety.

Regardless of your agreed management plan, you will need to agree with him a sensible **follow-up** interval. We would suggest that this is within the next 1–2 weeks.

As it is likely that you would be referring to adult social services, it is important to let the patient know what to expect and that they would be making contact very soon about arranging a visit. It may be worth considering arranging a joint visit with the daughter (and other family members if appropriate).

If the cough or chest signs persist, you should refer for a chest X-ray.

Further Reading

Action on Elder Abuse. http://www. elderabuse.org.uk/

Case C3

```
                        PATIENT

Name: Mr Dan de Souza
Age: 28
SH: Lives with partner in a shared 2-bed flat
PMH: Nil of note
DH: Nil
```

C3 Problem gambling

Patient brief: Mr Dan de Souza

You are a 28-year-old estate agent. You have come to see the doctor as you don't know who else to turn to. Over the past year you have changed from someone who enjoyed a '*little bet now and again*' to someone who is gambling recklessly and compulsively.

You have never told anybody about the extent of this problem and at times you may become quite emotional and tearful during the consultation.

It began when you and a friend opened up online poker playing accounts. At first this was quite fun and you would dip in and out of it. About a year ago you were given a promotion at work to become branch manager. The money was much better, but the stress level was higher and the hours were longer. This put a little strain on your relationship with your girlfriend, Emma. Around this time you started staying up late after Emma went to bed, playing poker online.

Initially you were gambling relatively small amounts, but this has increased over the year. Emma has no idea of the extent of this. About 6 months ago it got to the point where you were losing most of your disposable income. There have been many nights when you have stayed up all night '*chasing your losses*'. Things have been really bad over the last couple of months.

You had savings of £32,000 in a personal bank account that you were putting towards a deposit for a future home with Emma. You have gambled away all of this money. On one night alone recently you lost £5000. Emma does not know that you have lost this money. You had lied to her and told her that you would be investing it in shares. Last month you borrowed £1000 from a colleague at work and, having initially doubled your money to £2000, you had another 'all-nighter' after a stressful day and lost the lot. Nowadays when you start a gambling session you don't seem to be able to stop. You had to take out a payday loan to pay this month's rent.

You are under-performing at work, as you are often tired. You have been arguing a lot with Emma over '*silly things*'. You had a massive row last week. She feels that '*you don't give her any attention these days*' and that you don't respect her. She is threatening to leave. After the row, she walked out for a few days and, having had a week without gambling (which was tough), you then spent most of these 3 days playing poker online.

Increasingly you find you have little interest in the activities you used to enjoy (such as windsurfing) and you spend lots of time thinking about gambling.

You know that your gambling is out of control. Your life seems to be falling apart and you don't know who to turn to or what to do now. Your sleep is poor and you have started to hate yourself. If asked about suicidal thoughts, you will own up to having the idea sometimes that you would be better off dead, but you don't think you would act on this at the moment.

You don't take drugs. You drink alcohol socially. You have no previous psychiatric problems.

Patient's opening remarks: '*Doctor, I know this sounds weird but I think my life is getting kinda… out of control.*'

Patient's agenda: You want help to stop gambling. You have lost control. You don't know who to turn to for help.

EXAMINATION FINDINGS

Mental state well kempt and smart

Good eye contact

No obvious thought disorder

Low and tearful affect

No signs of deliberate self-harm (DSH)

Reflection

Key points

- **Data gathering:** Key areas are identifying features of addiction and the social impact of this problem.
- **Management:** You should offer appropriate options and give the patient ownership of the plan.

- **Interpersonal skills:** It is important to gather information in an open and non-judgemental manner. You should listen and respond to the patient's story.

Suggested marking criteria

	Clear Pass	Pass	Fail	Clear Fail
Data gathering	Gets a full picture of the story with a mix of predominantly open questions and skilful use of closed questioning only when necessary	Able to gather many of the features that are characteristic of addiction	Incomplete history (through ineffective active listening)	Fails to pick up impact of problem on the patient's life
Management	Patient has ownership of management plan and leaves with sense of hope	Explores options and gives patient opportunity to think these through and come up with own suggestions	Unstructured or unclear management options	Doctor not able to offer practical or worthwhile suggestions to patient
Interpersonal skills	Uncovers full picture of impact condition is having on patient's life	Respectful and gathers information through responding to patient's story	Interrupts flow of patient's story with excessive or early ICE questioning	Poor active listening or acts in clearly judgemental manner

Trainer's comments

Active listening with some simple encouragement should allow the majority of the important information to come out here. It is really important to allow this man time to talk. Through your data gathering, allow your patient to tell their story and talk about the impact it is having on their life. Do not interrupt too early and if you do ask questions, keep them open and relevant to what the patient is telling you. You are the first person this patient has opened up to. They have probably rehearsed what they are going to say to you. A strong candidate would be guided by **compassion and curiosity** and would not be distracted by ICE questions early in the data gathering.

If this has not been covered already, it is important that you enquire directly about the **impact the problem** gambling is having on this man's work and his relationship. Has anyone noticed his addiction: his partner, colleagues at work, his friends?

You would be expected to conduct this consultation in a **non-judgemental** manner.

You would be expected to **reflect back** to the patient that they have a gambling problem, ideally **in the language that they have used in the data-gathering** part of the consultation.

There are many features of problem gambling here (which mirror the features of any addiction), including:

- Gambling to the exclusion of other activities.
- Gambling compulsively and for long periods.
- Gambling having a significant impact on relationship/work.
- Covering up gambling and losses.
- Borrowing money to gamble.

There are several threads that you could explore in your **management plan**, such as:

- Referral to local addiction services (which would probably also have access to specialist gambling services).
- Signposting to voluntary-sector organisations (for example, Gamcare (1)) for support, information and advice.
- Signposting to local debt advice service.

You may want to use some motivational interviewing techniques to encourage some self-reflection about the potential gains of achieving change. For instance:

- 'How would your life be different if you stopped gambling?'
- 'What are the worst things that might happen if you don't make this change?'

You should definitely follow this patient up within the next month to assess progress and reassess risk.

Your plans for **follow-up** and **safety-netting** would need to be clear. Is it worth agreeing a joint consultation with his partner? Safety-netting should include a discussion around what to do in a crisis situation if any suicidal plans develop: for example, advice on out-of-hours services, A&E, any local emergency psychiatry provision or the Samaritans.

Reference

1. **Gamcare**: http://www.gamcare.org.uk

Further Reading

Royal College of Pyschiatrists. Problem gambling leaflet. http://www.rcpsych.ac.uk/healthadvice/problemsdisorders/problemgambling.aspx

Case C4

C4 Prostate Specific Antigen (PSA) test

Patient brief: Mr Glenmore Phillips

You are a 60-year-old market trader. You are coming to see the doctor as you are worried that you have prostate cancer. One of your friends from your local dominoes club has just been diagnosed with prostate cancer, and he has been advising you and the other guys to '*get the test*' (this was how his case was picked up).

This made you think about how you have been getting up to pass urine more often in the night (2–3 times most nights now) and how you sometimes have to rush to go during the day. Your stream is also slower than it used to be. This wasn't really bothering you much before (you thought it was just part of getting older, and you nip into the toilet in the café behind your stall when you need to), but when you spoke to your friend he said this was *exactly* how his cancer first presented itself, and he advised that you should *definitely* get the test.

You're not sure if you should be tested or not, so you want to talk this through with the doctor. If the doctor presents the pros and cons clearly to you, your instinct will be to go for the test. '*Better safe than sorry*,' you think.

There is no bleeding when passing urine, no appetite or weight loss, bowels normal. You are not excessively thirsty. You have no personal or family history of diabetes.

You have an uncle back in Jamaica who has 'prostate' – you're not sure if it is cancer or not.

You're not too keen on the idea of having a rectal examination, but if you feel relatively comfortable with the doctor then you will consent to this.

You like information to be presented clearly and will ask for things to be explained again if the doctor uses too much medical jargon.

Patient's opening remarks: '*My friend thinks I should get this "prostate test", doctor.*'

Patient's agenda: You are worried you may have prostate cancer and want to talk to the doctor about whether or not you should get the test. You have not made up your mind, but your instinct favours being tested.

You are not especially bothered by your symptoms of nocturia/urgency/poor stream and are not particularly interested in starting treatment for these.

EXAMINATION FINDINGS

Smoothly enlarged prostate
Urine dip clear
BP 136/85

Reflection

Key points

- **Data gathering:** Explore with curiosity and sensitivity.
- **Management:** A clear explanation delivered in manageable sections, along with checking understanding, is the foundation of a decision made in partnership with the patient.
- **Interpersonal skills:** Establish rapport with open consulting style. Communicate a complex area like this clearly, using language the patient understands.

Suggested marking criteria

	Clear Pass	Pass	Fail	Clear Fail
Data gathering	Gains clear understanding of patient's context and agenda	Gains clear understanding of symptoms and performs examination with sensitivity	Focuses excessively on LUTS rather than PSA query	Excessive probing for hidden agenda or hidden expectations that aren't there, to the point of frustrating the patient
Management	Patient is able to make decision in partnership with doctor having been active partner throughout consultation	Clear presentation of pros and cons of testing	Unable to communicate clearly that there are reasons for and against testing	Instructs patient on plan
Interpersonal skills	Delivers information clearly in small sections, checking understanding and summarising where necessary	Builds clear rapport with patient	Uses excessive medical jargon in explanation	Excessively paternalistic style, not involving the patient in consultation

Trainer's comments

This station will be a strong test of your **interpersonal skills**. While looking to build rapport and conduct the consultation with respect, you will be expected to demonstrate skills such as the ability to **communicate risks/benefits clearly** and to **make decisions in partnership** without exerting undue influence.

Data gathering should cover some key areas here. It's important to explore the patient's **risk factors** (specifically family history); he is already at increased risk from his Afro-Caribbean background (a threefold increase incidence compared to white males). It's also important to exclude other important conditions such as **diabetes** and **urinary tract infection**.

You should try to explore the patient's level of anxiety and reasons for asking for the test. This doesn't necessarily mean asking specific questions about his ideas, concerns and expectations (ICE). If you explore his agenda naturally, allowing the patient to talk, then these should arise naturally. Exploring what happened to his friend after the diagnosis is relevant, though: Did he require an operation? Has the cancer spread, is he worried about this?

As the patient has lower urinary tract symptoms (LUTS), a **digital rectal examination** would be appropriate. The patient is a little anxious about having this examination, so you should broach the subject with sensitivity and offer a chaperone. A urine dip test would also be appropriate. An opportunistic blood pressure check may be worthwhile, especially as he is at risk of having hypertension, being a middle-aged Afro-Caribbean man.

When it comes to **management,** remember that the PSA test has significant limitations. However, it is currently the best available test for identifying a localised prostate cancer (though, interestingly, it does not meet the standards for a population-based screening programme).

Offering a PSA test should include a balanced discussion with the patient about the potential benefits and limitations of the test. Potential benefits:

- It may be reassuring if the test is normal.
- It may lead to detection of cancer before symptoms develop.
- It may lead to detection of cancer at an early stage (for example, at a curable stage or when treatment could extend life).
- Test could be repeated in future, allowing monitoring of trend.

Limitations:

- It is not diagnostic. Further tests would be required for this: for example, transurethral resection of prostate (TURP), which carries its own risks of long-term complications such as incontinence and erectile dysfunction.
- It is not specific. Many other conditions increase the PSA level: for example, benign prostatic hyperplasia (BPH), urinary tract infection (UTI) and prostatitis. **About 2 in 3 men with a raised PSA will not have prostate cancer.**
- Many cases of prostate cancer do not cause an elevation of the PSA.

The Prostate Cancer Risk Management Programme quotes data showing that **15% of men with a normal PSA may have prostate cancer** (1).

- The test may lead to the diagnosis of cancers that may not have become apparent or shortened the patient's life.

An important GP skill is to be able to take complex information about pathology and risk and present this **clearly in language the patient understands**. The CSA examiners will be looking for this.

You would be expected to cover the above in manageable, bite-sized sections, **summarising** where appropriate and **checking the patient's understanding** regularly.

If you are going to arrange for a PSA test, it is important to remind the patient of some practicalities. Your patient should not have:

- An active UTI.
- Had a digital rectal examination in the last week.
- Have ejaculated or exercised vigorously in the last 48 hours (1).

If you are aware of a **patient information leaflet**, this may be used as a guide to decision making. Examples would be the (excellent) patient information leaflet on PSA testing from the Prostate Cancer Risk Management Programme (2) or the similar leaflet from patient.co.uk.

Lower urinary tract symptoms are much more likely to be caused by **benign prostatic hyperplasia (BPH)** than prostate cancer. Prostate cancers tend to be asymptomatic in both localised and locally advanced stages. This is because (in contrast to BPH) they most commonly arise in the outer portion of the prostate gland (1).

You could offer simple advice on conservative measures (for example, reduced caffeine and alcohol intake) and explore the option of medical treatment for these symptoms, but **do not push this if the patient is not interested**.

Opportunistic **screening for diabetes** may also be appropriate (this patient is at high risk given his age and his Afro-Caribbean background).

References

1. Prostate Cancer Risk Management Programme. Information for primary care. http://www.cancerscreening.nhs.uk/prostate/prostate-booklet-text.pdf
2. Public Health England. Prostate Cancer Risk Management Programme. http://www.cancerscreening.nhs.uk/prostate/informationpack.html

Case C5

PATIENT
Name: Ms Sahra Osman
Age: 23
SH: Born in Somalia, moved to UK with family to flee civil war aged 9
Lives with parents and 3 younger siblings
No smoking/alcohol
PMH: UTI x 3 in last 2 years
DH: Nil

C5 Female Genital Mutilation (FGM)

Patient brief: Ms Sahra Osman

You are a 23-year-old GP's receptionist. Over the past couple of years you have been experiencing increasing symptoms of urinary incontinence. This has happened to some degree for as long as you can remember (after coughing or laughing), but increasingly it is happening at random and with less warning. Often you can get to the bathroom in time, although this not always the case. There have been a couple of incidents in the last two months that have made you feel particularly ashamed. One was when you were working on the front desk at the surgery on a busy Monday morning. The other was in the queue for a changing room. On both occasions you were incontinent of urine; both times you think you were just about able to hide this.

Also when you pass urine the stream is slow and for as long as you remember you have to push to empty your bladder completely.

When you were 7 you experienced what you refer to as 'the cut' (female circumcision/female genital mutilation). This was a frightening experience and something you never talk about. After seeing a poster in the practice you did some reading online and you think that this procedure may have caused your problems.

You are engaged to be married and your fiancé is also from the local Somali community. You are very worried about having intercourse with your husband because of the effect of 'the cut'. You are afraid that permanent damage may have been done. You have never had intercourse.

You menstruate regularly, bleeding for 4 days in a 28-day cycle. Your periods have always been painful, more so over the last 2 years.

You have never talked about any of this to a healthcare professional, but you have come prepared to talk today. However, it won't be easy. If you are given space and feel listened to (and the doctor shows you respect), you will open up. You will explain that you have had 'the cut' and talk more about your fears that it may have damaged you.

You are not prepared to be examined today. Even if you feel you can trust the doctor, you will not allow an examination. You ideally would like to be referred to 'the specialist' without being examined – and then they can examine you. If pushed, you will say you are menstruating today. If you really feel you can trust the doctor then you may consent to book in for another appointment on another day for examination.

If the doctor refuses to take the consultation further without examination, then you will burst into tears.

If the doctor is struggling to understand what 'the cut' is, you should explain that it's female circumcision.

Patient's opening remarks. '*I'm having problems passing urine all the time. I think I need to see a specialist.*'

Patient's agenda: You have experienced FGM as a child and are worried about:
- The effect it has had on your urinary continence.
- The effect it may have on your upcoming marriage. You are very apprehensive about your future sexual relationship.

You are clear that you want to see a gynaecologist to get this problem sorted out.

EXAMINATION FINDINGS
Does not consent to examination.

Reflection
Key points
- **Data gathering:** Use active listening and sensitive encouragement to allow the patient to tell her story. If this doesn't happen easily, then you will need to cover a more structured urological/gynaecological and social history.

- **Management:** Onward referral would be appropriate even in the absence of examination.

- **Interpersonal skills:** It is vital that you listen to the patient and treat her with respect. She needs to feel that she can trust the doctor – only then will she tell the full story about her FGM. This will require active listening and picking up on cues.

Suggested marking criteria

	Clear Pass	Pass	Fail	Clear Fail
Data gathering	Gains clear understanding of physical and psychological impact of FGM, especially around fears with future relationship	Following allowing the patient to talk, 'fills the gaps' in data gathering without duplication	Limited exploration of FGM	Does not pick up patient has had FGM
Management	Explains clearly and uses patient's understanding in explanation; refers appropriately to specialist	Patient involved in management plan; refers appropriately to specialist	Unclear or inappropriate management plan	Will not proceed without examination; excessively doctor-centred about this
Interpersonal skills	Treats patient with warmth and respect; patient trusts the doctor and feels she has been listened to and treated appropriately	Responds to cues	Fails to pick up worries over future relationship	Uses excessive medical jargon

Trainer's comments

Interpersonal skills are central here: this is a case that should be approached with sensitivity and respect. It is only if the patient feels she can trust the doctor that she will open up with the deeper levels of her story, its impact and her fears. The doctor should show warmth and openness. Active listening, responding to cues and giving the patient space to talk are all essential here. She will not respond well to interruption or excessive medical jargon. You should express yourself clearly and sensitively, drawing on the patient's knowledge and understanding.

Don't miss the key issue here (FGM) – it is important that you gain a good understanding of the urological/gynaecological picture, but this is a case where the examiners will be just as interested to see how you manage the exploration of FGM and its impact.

It is really important that you gain a clear understanding of **the impact of her symptoms** on her life so far and her fears for the future (notably with respect to her engagement to be married). This should be done with sensitivity.

FGM **is illegal** in the UK; this should be clarified and could be explored further. What are her views on it? Are any siblings, other family members or friends similarly affected? What about her thoughts when she has children?

Respect the patient's autonomy – her reluctance to be examined should definitely not be pushed. Her keenness to see a specialist seems reasonable and should be respected. There is a risk that if you ask her to re-book for an examination, she may not return.

Your **management** should include referral to a specialist gynaecology service. You should give her an outline of what may be offered: for instance, surgical procedures to address symptoms and reverse some of the damage. You may also want to consider onward referral to psychological services or voluntary-sector/support services.

It would be good to discuss what follow-up arrangements you would like to put in place (for example, review after clinic). It is worth being aware that this woman would benefit from a trusting, ongoing relationship with her GP as she navigates her future treatment. **Relationship building** is key here.

FGM is a common practice in East and Central Africa. According to UNICEF (1), the top rates are in Somalia (98% of women affected), Guinea (96%), Djibouti (93%), Egypt (91%), Eritrea (89%), Mali (89%), Sierra Leone (88%), Sudan (88%), Gambia (76%), Burkina Faso (76%), Ethiopia (74%), Mauritania (69%), Liberia (66%) and Guinea-Bissau (50%). It is estimated that over 20,000 girls under the age of 15 are at risk of FGM in the UK each year, and that 66,000 women in the UK have had FGM. However, the true extent of the problem is unknown (2).

FGM can lead to a variety of long-term urological/gynaecological complications, including recurrent infections, incontinence, difficulty voiding and dyspareunia, as well as psychological damage, including flashbacks, depression and low libido (2).

References

1. UNICEF. Female genital mutilation/ 'Cutting' – a statistical overview and exploration of the dynamics of change. http://www.unicef.org/media/files/FGCM_Lo_res.pdf
2. NHS information on FGM. www.nhs.uk/Conditions/female-genital-mutilation/

Further Reading

FGM: Multi-agency practice guidelines. https://www.gov.uk/government/publications/female-genital-mutilation-multi-agency-practice-guidelines

World Health Organisation (WHO) factsheet on FGM. http://www.who.int/mediacentre/factsheets/fs241/en/

Case C6

PATIENT

Name: Mr Peter Atkinson

Age: 57

SH: Long-standing smoker. Cut down from 40 to 10 per day over the last couple of years.

PMH: COPD diagnosed 5 years ago. No spirometry for the past 3 years.

DH: The below are listed on **repeat medication** list. All appear to be under-used. None of these has been issued for the past six months:

Salbutamol 100 mcg inhaler – 2 puffs qds prn

Tiotropium 18 mcg inhaler – one puff od

Fluticasone 125 mcg/salmeterol 25 mcg inhaler – 2 puffs bd

C6 COPD exacerbation

Patient brief: Mr Peter Atkinson

You are a 57-year-old electrician and you have come to see the doctor because you have had a cough over the last 3 weeks that you can't seem to shift. It is usual for you to cough up a little clear phlegm in the morning (your 'smoker's cough'), but you are now coughing throughout the day and the phlegm is thicker and yellow-tinged.

You usually get a 'chest infection' once a year and this tends to respond well to antibiotics. You would like to get some antibiotics and get on your way; *'We're both busy people'*.

Your breathing has been unchanged from your normal levels – you tend to get short of breath when walking up stairs or walking about 50 metres. This is not something you will bring up unless directly asked as you think this is *'normal for someone with bronchitis'*.

It's not really part of your plan for the consultation to talk much about your chronic obstructive pulmonary disease (COPD), so this will need some encouragement from the doctor. However, if you like the doctor and he or she treats you with respect, you will respond to any questions.

You have a very sketchy understanding of COPD. You know that it's something to do with smoking and that it makes you cough. You take your blue inhaler on an 'as and when' basis. You take your other inhalers erratically. You're not really clear when you should take them or even whether they work or not. You might try to cover this up a little in front of the doctor if you don't feel like you can trust them. You're not someone to trouble the doctor.

You get three or four coughs every winter – you usually need antibiotics to shift a couple of them. You've never been offered pulmonary rehabilitation, as far as you can recall.

There's no history of weight loss, chest pain or haemoptysis, no asbestos exposure that you know of (though having worked as an electrician for most of your life, you can't rule it out) and no recent foreign travel.

You have smoked since you were 14. For many years you smoked 40 a day. You tried stopping (without medical help) 5 years ago as a New Year resolution. This was after one of your friends from the local darts team died of lung cancer. You don't see the point of '*patches, or any of that rubbish*' and your attitude is that it's '*all about willpower*'. You have cut down to 10 a day over the last few years.

You are a proud and slightly stubborn man and you will not respond well to being talked down to by the doctor. You would be responsive to working with a doctor who treats you with respect.

If the doctor suggests a chest X-ray you will wonder whether it's really necessary.

If the doctor mentions cancer you will be shocked into seriousness: '*Do you think it's cancer, doc?*'

Patient's opening remarks: '*I think I need my "once-a-year antibiotics" for my chest, doc.*'

Patient's agenda: You want some antibiotics for what you consider to be a chest infection. You suspect this should clear things up. You know you really should stop smoking.

EXAMINATION FINDINGS

Temperature 36.9 °C
Pulse 88 regular
BP 118/78
Respiratory rate 16
Oxygen saturation 96%
Chest – bilateral mild wheeze throughout
No clubbing
No cervical lymphadenopathy
Peak flow 330 l/min

Reflection

Key points

- **Data gathering:** Cover red flags, acute presentation, chronic condition (including the patient's lack of understanding and the impact of the condition) and smoking history.
- **Management:** Cover acute presentation, chronic condition and health promotion.
- **Interpersonal skills:** You need to strike a balance here between respecting the patient's agenda and exploring his lack of understanding and engagement. This should be done in a respectful and non-judgemental manner.

Suggested marking criteria

	Clear Pass	Pass	Fail	Clear Fail
Data gathering	Picks up that there may be an element of denial in the patient's lack of understanding	Achieves understanding of acute and chronic picture with mix of open and closed questions	Incomplete history (especially with respect to ongoing COPD symptoms) or examination	Misses red flags (e.g. smoking history)
Management	Works with patient to agree a plan that covers other areas such as pulmonary rehab and reviewing inhaler technique; patient has ownership of plan	Both treats acute presentation and involves practice team appropriately in long-term management	Treats acute presentation without tackling chronic management or the patient's lack of understanding; no clear follow-up plan	No plans for chest X-ray
Interpersonal skills	Uses reflective questioning to encourage change	Treats patient with respect and gains information sensitively, especially with respect to the patient's lack of understanding of his condition	Does not pick up on patient's knowledge that he should stop smoking	Talks down to the patient or makes him feel stupid

Trainer's comments

You need to address important **red flags** (1):

- **Urgent chest X-ray**: As there is a significant change in symptoms in someone with established COPD (and a lifelong smoker), an urgent chest X-ray needs to be considered. It could be offered now or after treatment of this infective exacerbation of COPD.

Either way, it is important that you discuss this.

- **Possible persisting haemoptysis:** Smokers presenting with haemoptysis should be referred on the 2-week rule regardless of chest X-ray, so enquire directly about this.

This consultation will require a skilful balance. The patient's agenda is predominantly focused on the acute presentation; however, you should also be looking at the chronic condition. To achieve this it is essential that the patient feels you respect him and that you are working with him in this consultation. It is important that you establish a **rapport** with the patient as early as possible in the consultation.

Data gathering should cover the acute presentation, red flags (for example, haemoptysis, weight loss), the chronic picture (for example, breathing, frequency of exacerbations), understanding of condition (or lack of it), impact on life and smoking history. There is a lot to cover here. It's important that you don't waste time asking unnecessary questions or putting the same question twice. You should consider assessment or subsequent review of inhaler technique.

In terms of **management** within the consultation, the examiners would expect you to tackle the following three main areas, as well as taking into account the patient's health beliefs and what he expects from the consultation:

- **Manage the acute presentation.** A chest X-ray would be expected either now or after treatment if still symptomatic, as would a course of antibiotics (as per current local guidelines) and oral steroids.

- **Manage the chronic health problem**. This hinges on the patient's lack of understanding, which you should aim to address with a **clear explanation** of COPD that **reflects the patient's own language and understanding**. A patient information leaflet may be helpful here if you are aware of one (for example, from patient.co.uk), but this is only as an adjunct to a good explanation. It may be worth arranging follow-up with the practice nurse who could explore inhaler technique and a treatment regime that is in line with the 2010 NICE guidance (2). A referral to pulmonary rehabilitation should be offered. Practise how to explain what pulmonary rehabilitation is. There are some very good YouTube videos about this that might help your explanation.

- **Engage in health promotion (stopping smoking)**. You should definitely be looking to assess the patient's readiness to change and offering smoking cessation advice. Good candidates would use **reflective questions to enable change**. **Motivational interviewing** techniques can be used to achieve this in a consultation. For instance:
  - 'What would be the best things that would happen if you stopped smoking?'
  - 'If you were successful in stopping smoking, what would be different?'

The examiners would expect you to **be realistic**. There are certain things you must do in this consultation (for example, treat an exacerbation; consider your plans for chest X-ray; explore the patient's lack of understanding; offer smoking-cessation advice); however, it is reasonable to continue this management at a later date with yourself or another member of the team (for example, the practice nurse). It is really important that you are seen to be **working with the patient** throughout the consultation.

You will also need to consider your plans for **follow-up** and how to approach **safety-netting** for this patient. For instance: 'I would expect that with this treatment you should be better by the end of the course. But if you are still coughing or are short of breath then you should come back to see me. Also, if things deteriorate significantly with your breathing, it's important you seek medical advice.'

References

1. National Institute for Health and Clinical Excellence (2011) *Referral Guidelines for Suspected Cancer*. London: NICE. http://guidance.nice. org.uk/CG27
2. National Institute for Health and Clinical Excellence (2010) *Management of Chronic Obstructive Pulmonary Disease (COPD) in Adults in Primary and Secondary Care*. London: NICE. http://guidance.nice.org.uk/CG101

Case C7

PATIENT

Name: Mr James McGregor
Age: 32
SH: Lives alone, non-smoker, moderate alcohol
PMH: Nil of note

Took HIV test as part of new patient health check (performed by the healthcare assistant, HCA). Returning to see GP for results.

Blood test result
Serum HIV – positive

C7 Blood test results HIV positive

Patient brief: Mr James McGregor

You are a 32-year-old civil servant and you have booked in to see the doctor to get the results from your recent HIV test.

If the doctor starts asking you lots of questions before giving you the result, you will become a little frustrated and will ask directly for the result.

You are prepared to talk about your sexual history if asked, and will be more comfortable if the doctor seems comfortable and confident. You last had an HIV test 2 years ago, at the beginning of your most recent relationship. This was with the local sexual health clinic.

You are a gay man and you have been in a stable relationship with your partner Carlos (37) over the past 2 years. You both had (negative) HIV tests at the start of your relationship. You practise (unprotected) anal intercourse and you are the receptive partner. You and your partner have an understanding that any intercourse outside of the relationship must be protected. You have had 2 casual partners over the past 6 months (protected anal intercourse and unprotected oral intercourse). You suspect your partner may have had more, and recently you have been arguing quite a lot.

When the healthcare assistant offered you the test at registration, you had a sense that it was worth doing. Carlos does not know you took the test.

You have a couple of friends who are HIV positive. One is a man your age and one is a man in his 50s. They both seem reasonably healthy. The man in his 50s has mild arthritis. You know that the outlook for HIV is better than it used to be and that there is now medication for HIV that works quite well.

When you are told of your HIV status you are very upset, but not completely surprised.

You have never used any intravenous drugs. You drink only at the weekends.

You do not suffer from recurrent infections and have no significant weight loss.

Patient's opening remarks: '*I've come to get the results of my HIV test, doctor.*'

Patient's agenda: You want to know your test result. You have a hunch that it may be positive.

EXAMINATION FINDINGS

No palpable lymphadenopathy

Reflection

Key points

- **Data gathering:** It is important to explore the patient's understanding and the psychosocial context.

- **Management:** Explanation and plan should be clearly expressed and incorporate the patient's understanding.

- **Interpersonal skills:** You should demonstrate an open and non-judgemental approach.

Suggested marking criteria

	Clear Pass	Pass	Fail	Clear Fail
Data gathering	Flow of data gathering is natural and comfortable, and uses patient's understanding to frame explanations	Clarifies patient's understanding of HIV and experiences of HIV	Inadequate grasp of psychosocial context	Didactic approach to data gathering (for example, will not tell patient results until full sexual history completed)
Management	Uses patient's understanding in explaining diagnosis, prognosis and future treatment	Expresses diagnosis clearly in non-medical jargon	Unclear follow-up or future plans; not clear on contact tracing	Offers patient inappropriate management options in misguided attempt at offering choice
Interpersonal skills	Establishes comfortable rapport, confidence with flow of consultation not following usual 'CSA structure'; patient would see doctor again	Conducts consultation with emotional warmth and respect; non-judgemental	Rushes patient (especially when taking in the diagnosis)	Judgemental in approach

Trainer's comments

This case shows how you need to be flexible in your approach to what a CSA case 'looks like'. If you try to follow the classic structure (i.e. Data gathering → Explanation → Management plan), then you are likely to run into trouble. You need to be able to be confident in managing the structure flexibly in a consultation like this, probably starting with an explanation and then flowing between explanation, data gathering and management.

There are three tasks that you need to achieve at the beginning of the consultation:

- **Communicate the results of the test**. Do not at this point go into extensive data-gathering mode. If you spend time here collecting a sexual history and asking your ICE questions before communicating the result, you will frustrate the patient. His agenda is clear – he has come for the test result.

- **Explain the diagnosis**. As with all explanations, these work best when framed by the patient's understanding. It would be a good idea to explore this with the patient before beginning your explanation. Good questions may be 'What do you know about HIV?' or 'Do you know anyone who has HIV' or 'Do you know why the test was done?'. This will then guide your explanation. It may be that your patient has a pretty good understanding of the condition already. This is the crux of the consultation and it is really important not to rush this. You should

check understanding and you should give the patient plenty of opportunity to ask you questions about this diagnosis. You need to be responsive to the **emotional impact** of the diagnosis. Give the patient time to take this in.

- **Establish rapport with the patient**. Throughout these initial exchanges you should look to build rapport with the patient. You must maintain an open and non-judgemental manner.

It would be worth exploring his relationship issues. What support is in place if the relationship breaks up as a result of the diagnosis? Are there friends and family he can speak to? What about the impact on work?

Is his partner a patient of yours? Are there confidentiality issues? It would be good to confirm with your patient if he intends to discuss the result with his partner.

You may find that directing the patient to a website such as the Terrence Higgins Trust (1) would be a helpful source for further information about this new diagnosis.

You should feel comfortable with allowing the flow of the consultation to follow the patient, but you should look to include:

- **A discussion on prognosis and treatment** shaped by the patient's understanding, which you should ask about directly. You need to find the right balance here (communicating that the majority of people with HIV live long and healthy lives) without offering false reassurance.

- **Planning next steps**. You should communicate that you will be referring to a specialist HIV team, and again allow for any questions. It is likely that you will need to repeat the test, although most of the time it is very reliable.
- **A sexual history and exploration of your patient's current state of health**. You should be flexible about when feels the right time to gather a **sexual history** and to ask directly about intravenous drug use. This would then guide your advice about **contact tracing**, which would most likely be overseen by the specialist team. It is important that you conduct this in an open, non-judgemental manner. You will also need to consider **screening for other sexually transmitted infections**.

In terms of **follow-up**, although the specialist team will take the lead on the management of this man's condition, you will, as his GP, be involved in his long-term care (of both his HIV and any other conditions). It is important to communicate this. If this consultation has been conducted with sensitivity and respect, then this will lay a foundation for a good doctor–patient relationship.

Reference
1. Terrence Higgins Trust. http://www.tht.org.uk/

Further Reading
NICE Clinical Knowledge Summaries. Guidance on HIV infection and AIDS. http://cks.nice.org.uk/hiv-infection-and-aids

Case C8

C8 Breast lump (learning disability)

Patient brief: Miss Susan ('Sue') Owen

You are a 58-year-old woman and you do voluntary work in a local charity shop twice a week (helping sort new donations). You have come to see the doctor because the other day you told Janet (your warden and friend) that you had noticed 'something funny' in your right breast – it is a hard lump. You don't know what it is but it doesn't seem right. Janet said it was best to make an appointment to see the doctor. You agreed this was a good idea and you let Janet book this for you.

You have no idea what the lump is. There has been nothing else going on. There is no bleeding; no nipple discharge or skin change that you have noticed; no appetite change/weight loss. There is no family history of breast problems that you know about.

You are very shy around people you don't know well, especially doctors. You spent a week in hospital with pneumonia a few years ago. It was a noisy and frightening experience.

At the beginning of the consultation you are not ready to talk about yourself and will spend the first minute or two asking the doctor to have a look at 'Peggy', as she has a tummy ache.

If the doctor seems nice you will talk to them and become less shy. If the doctor seems stern then you will look down at your shoes and play with 'Peggy'.

You are shy about being examined, although less so if the doctor uses 'Peggy' to show you what happens during the examination. If you are feeling shy around the doctor it would help if they were nice to 'Peggy'.

Even though you have a low IQ, you are capable of understanding what is going on if it is expressed in clear and simple terms, and you are likewise capable of making decisions about things. You don't mind letting the doctor make the decision for you if they seem nice and sensible.

When the doctor says you might have to go to a hospital clinic you will look very sad and hug 'Peggy' for support. You are worried that they will keep you in like last time.

The only person you know who had cancer was your friend Ray from your home. He died. You don't know what cancer he had.

Patient's opening remarks: *'Hello, doctor. This is Peggy and I am Sue. Peggy is not well today.'*

Patient's agenda: There is no hidden agenda here. You are simply here because Janet said it was best to see the doctor about what you have noticed in your breast.

EXAMINATION FINDINGS

Right breast: a hard craggy 2 cm lump deep to left of areola

No lymphadenopathy

No nipple changes/discharge

No skin changes

Other breast NAD

Reflection

Key points

- **Data gathering:** It's important that this is as natural as possible. Aggressive, interrogative questioning may cause the relationship to break down, as could rushing the patient. You need to assess the patient's capacity to consent to examination and to understand management.

- **Management:** It is important that the patient is involved here.

- **Interpersonal skills:** You must establish trust. This would be helped by communicating kindness and sensitivity, as well as expressing yourself clearly. The doll may be a useful tool here.

Suggested marking criteria

	Clear Pass	Pass	Fail	Clear Fail
Data gathering	Addresses her fear of hospitals with sensitivity	Gathers information in a natural, sensitive style	Does not give patient time to express herself clearly	Confuses patient with aggressive ICE questions
Management	Refers appropriately to clinic, with patient feeling like she was involved in making this decision	Refers appropriately under the '2-week rule', with patient understanding why and what will happen next and with clear plan for follow-up	Patient does not really understand management plan and potential seriousness of condition	Does not refer under the '2-week rule'
Interpersonal skills	Delivers information clearly, summarising and checking understanding	Conducts consultation with sensitivity and respect	Rushes patient or fails to build relationship; patient not sure if she would see the doctor again	Loses patient with medical jargon

Trainer's comments

One of the key things the examiners will be looking for here is your ability to build a **trusting relationship** with this patient during the consultation. Communicating kindness and sensitivity is key here, as is giving her time to trust you. Her doll 'Peggy' may be a useful tool to gain her trust. Sue will not respond well to a succession of standard 'ICE' questions. **Building trust** is more important than digging for a hidden agenda that does not exist or uncovering expectations that are not there.

You need to be confident that Sue has the **capacity** to consent to examination and to understand her management. The Mental Capacity Act 2005 (3) states that mental capacity is the ability to make decisions for yourself. To demonstrate capacity an individual needs to be able to:

• **Understand information**
• **Retain the information** long enough to be able to make the decision
• **Weigh up the information** to make the decision
• **Communicate their decision**

The examiners might well be asking themselves: 'Would this patient see this doctor again?' It is vital that this feels like a natural, warm consultation.

Sue will need a clear explanation, free from any medical jargon. It would be very valuable to check understanding (in a way that feels natural) here and when discussing the management plan.

Try to **involve Sue in her management plan** – this will require you to be clear, to give her time and to summarise information when necessary. This presentation would meet the 2-week rule for suspected cancer (2). It is important to be clear to Sue what to expect next and to mention clearly that this is a referral to **exclude cancer**, **checking that she understands** that this is important.

Under the NICE 2-week guidance you should urgently refer patients using the following criteria:

- Any age with a suspected malignant lump
- Aged 25+ with a change in texture of the breast perceived by the patient
- With a history of breast cancer who presents with a further lump or suspicious symptoms
- With unilateral eczematous nipple change that does not respond to topical treatment
- With nipple distortion of recent onset (not retractile nipple)
- With spontaneous unilateral blood-stained or serous nipple discharge
- With unexplained inflammatory changes (erythema and skin oedema)
- Who are male, aged 50 years and older with a unilateral subareolar mass with or without nipple distortion or associated skin changes

Do not offer false reassurance; you have a duty to be **honest** to the patient and to tell her that a hospital outpatient attendance and biopsy are likely. Admission for surgery in the future could not be ruled out. Ensuring that she has capacity for an examination would be important. Can she understand, process and retain the information you give her, while conveying her decision? If so, then she has capacity.

In terms of **follow-up**, if Sue does turn out to have breast cancer (as seems likely) then she will benefit from a trusting relationship with her GP. She is bound to have some questions after attending clinic, so a review a couple of weeks after then would be sensible. She may well have some unanswered questions.

References

1. Mental Capacity Act 2005. http://www.legislation.gov.uk/ukpga/2005/9/contents
2. National Institute for Health and Clinical Excellence (2011) *Referral Guidelines for Suspected Cancer*. London: NICE. http://guidance.nice.org.uk/CG27

PATIENT

Name: Mr David Cooke

Age: 56

PMH: 8 weeks post **partial thyroidectomy** for benign cyst. Some bleeding post-op (stayed in overnight). 2 weeks post-op saw a GP, who signed him off for 6 weeks. 6 weeks post-op seen in surgical outpatients.

Brief letter scanned in notes, mentions post-op bleed, but now making 'solid recovery'. No comment on return to work. Thyroid function normal.

C9 Request for sick note

Patient brief: Mr David Cooke

You are a 56-year-old delivery driver. You have come to see the doctor today because you need to get your sick note extended for another 6 weeks so you can make a 'full recovery' from your recent surgery. You were signed off previously by one of the senior doctors in the practice – according to you '*they know what they're talking about*'.

You do not want to talk in any detail about your condition. If the doctor asks why you need another 6 weeks off, you will say it is all in the notes and that you've just had '*major surgery for a lump in your neck*'.

You are annoyed that you always seem to see a different doctor at this practice: '*I'm fed up that I have to keep starting from square one. Dr Williams signed me off, she knows what she's doing.*'

You are adamant that the surgeon has told you that you should take as much time as you need to recover.

You think that the doctor seems very young and you will comment on this: '*You must be only about 20, doctor. You don't know what it's really like out there.*' You don't trust the new doctors in the practice as much as the experienced doctors.

If the doctor presses you to talk more in a way that you feel is aggressive, you will get angry and bang your fist and say: '*Just give me the sick note.*'

Later in the consultation, if you feel comfortable to talk you will open up that you are worried that when you turn your head driving or when you do some lifting then the scar may open up and you may bleed again. If this happens on the road then you are worried that this is could be dangerous.

Patient's opening remarks: '*I just need another sick note, doctor.*'

Patient's agenda: You need a sick note, and this young doctor probably doesn't know what they are talking about. You are also worried about the scar opening up and bleeding when you drive.

> ## EXAMINATION FINDINGS
> Well-healed post-operative scar.

Reflection
Key points

- **Data gathering:** You should respond to the patient's story and explore further with open questions.
- **Management:** This should be appropriate (there is more information in the trainer's comments) and you should draw on the patient's health beliefs and agenda when discussing this.
- **Interpersonal skills:** Adopt a calm approach, with open body language. Listen to the patient, responding to cues.

Suggested marking criteria

	Clear Pass	Pass	Fail	Clear Fail
Data gathering	Data gathering is selective and appropriate	Clear history of post-op complications and of patient's health beliefs, especially with reference to worries about wound 'opening up'	Does not address why patient thinks he needs 6 weeks further off work	Unable to get clear picture from data gathering as consultation descends into argument
Management	Is able to agree plans for a return to work with terms that are appropriate, and with the patient taking an active role in this decision	Explores return to work, considering graded return; agrees appropriate follow-up plans	Inadequately explores options of shorter duration of sick note or of graded return to work	Issues 6-week sick note without question
Interpersonal skills	Is able to engage with patient on equal adult–adult footing; patient would come back to see this doctor	Listens to patient with open body language; responsive to patient's agenda and health beliefs, especially with reference to worries about wound 'opening up'	No exploration of context (especially with reference to work)	Loses temper with patient; interrupts patient

Trainer's comments

The key challenges for this case are:

- Dealing with a request for a sick note that may not be appropriate
- Dealing with a patient who is seeking to gain the upper hand in the consultation through putting the doctor down

This case may seem a little daunting at first, but as ever, success hinges on good **interpersonal skills** and **data gathering**.

It is easy to feel quite affronted or annoyed if a patient seems to be trying to put you down to gain the upper hand. You should recognise that this is happening and use good interpersonal skills to re-negotiate the dynamic of the consultation.

It might be helpful in these cases to remember the ideas of '**Transactional Analysis**' developed by Eric Berne in the 1960s (1). Berne describes three states:

- **Parent**
- **Adult**
- **Child**

The healthy 'patient-centred' consultation should aim for an **Adult–Adult** dynamic.

Paternalistic consultations may lead to a **Parent–Child** dynamic, with the doctor wielding power over the patient. Sometimes patients may draw the doctor into this kind of interaction: for example, by adopting a **Child**-like role when they are keen on passing responsibility over to the doctor.

This consultation is an example of where the patient is adopting a **Parent–**

Child dynamic (with the patient as **Parent** and doctor as **Child**). The doctor should aim to normalise this power dynamic to an **Adult–Adult** interaction with good interpersonal skills, specifically in this case:

- Maintain a **calm and non-judgemental manner** throughout.
- Maintain **open body language**.
- Do not get drawn into an argument.
- **Listen** to the patient, allowing him to outline his story.
- Explore with **open questions**.
- **Pick up cues** that may help you uncover the patient's health beliefs and agenda.

Taking this approach in a calm and confident manner should stand you in good stead when you move on to your management plan. If the patient has been **listened** to and their story has been **explored confidently and with respect**, you should be in a strong position to proceed to your clinical management on an equal footing.

In this case you need to earn the patient's respect through your professionalism. The trap to avoid would be to be drawn into a '**Child–Child**' interaction: for instance, if you point-blank refuse medical certification or accuse the patient of trying to falsify his claim for a further medical certification. This could lead the consultation to deteriorate into a highly dysfunctional **Child–Child** interaction.

Your **clinical management** should be appropriate. It would be wrong to offer the patient a further 6 weeks' certification. Your discussion should:

- Draw on the **patient's health belief** that returning to work too early may be damaging to him.
- **Agree a plan for a return to work**. You may explore a graded return to work or reviewing the patient again after a short timeframe (for example, 1–2 weeks). When presenting your ideas for management (for example, plans for future certification), you should be clear in your justification. Remember, when you agree that the patient is fit to work, the fitness to work certificate allows you to specify particular conditions (for example, amended duties or a phased return to work) if certain activities are problematic (such as turning his head).

The company may be able to suggest some alternative work: for example, in the office rather than driving.

You should agree clear follow-up plans with the patient. If the consultation has gone well, this follow-up should be with you.

Reference

1. Berne, E. (2010) *Games People Play: The Psychology of Human Relationships*. Harmondsworth: Penguin.

Further Reading

Royal College of Surgeons. Get well soon: Helping you make a speedy recovery after a thyroidectomy. http://www.rcseng.ac.uk/patients/get-well-soon/thyroidectomy/

Case C10

PATIENT

Name: Miss Ayofemi Akintola

Age: 17

Occupation: At college studying A-Levels

SH: Lives at home with parents and two brothers. She is the middle child.

PMH: Sickle cell disease. Annual follow-up in specialist haematology clinic (last seen 18 months ago, but has not attended on last two occasions). Only previous crisis was at 12 years of age, requiring admission.

FH: Both parents and both siblings have sickle cell trait

DH: Penicillin V 500 mg bd (112 tablets) on repeat list – has not been requested for 4 months

There is an alert on the system to say she is due annual flu vaccination and pneumovax booster. She missed last year's flu jab.

C10 Sickle cell (adolescent)

Patient brief: Miss Ayofemi Akintola

You are just recovering from a nasty cold. Yesterday you had netball practice, followed straight afterwards by a competitive match. Your team won, but it was a tough game and it was freezing outside. You woke up early today with pain in both legs (between your hips and knees) and a slight temperature. Your mum has booked you an appointment to see the doctor. You told her you would prefer to see the doctor on your own.

You feel it is unfair that you have sickle cell disease; your brothers don't have it.

You missed your last two clinic appointments because they clashed with a school trip and a netball game, and you haven't got round to booking your next appointment with the clinic yet. Previously you had always attended clinic regularly with mum.

You've been really busy recently with school; you got ten A* grades at GCSE and you are working hard at college now. You are applying to study medicine. You are also a key player in the school netball team.

If asked sensitively, you will own up to missing quite a few of your penicillin tablets. If the doctor is insensitive, you will try to cover this up by saying that you had some 'stored up from before'.

You have not got round to getting your flu jab yet this winter.

You do not usually get sickle cell crises and you are not in regular pain.

If asked, your periods are regular and your menarche was at 13 years old.

You have had a boyfriend for 2 years – you are currently not sexually active.

Patient's opening remarks: '*I'm feeling really ill, doctor, and my legs are hurting.*'

Patient's agenda: You don't know if this is just 'aches and pains' after a big game or if you are having a crisis. You have been 'too busy' to think about your sickle cell disease recently. There is an element of denial here.

EXAMINATION FINDINGS

Temperature 38.4 °C

Pulse 92 regular

BP 108/68

Hips and knee: both full range of movement, generalised pain just above both knees bilaterally

Chest: clear

Abdomen: Soft, no hepato- or splenomegaly

Reflection

Key points

- **Data gathering:** You should cover the acute presentation, long-term condition, patient's understanding and the effect (both physical and psychological) of the illness.

- **Management:** A good candidate would use reflective questioning to help the patient take ownership of the management of her long-term condition.

- **Interpersonal skills:** You should connect with the patient enough to engage her without being patronising, while still challenging her appropriately.

Suggested marking criteria

	Clear Pass	Pass	Fail	Clear Fail
Data gathering	Achieves clear understanding of reasons for disengagement and the impact of the diagnosis on the patient as a person	Achieves clear understanding of details of acute presentation and long-term condition	Does not adequately explore engagement with long-term condition	Unfocused or incomplete examination
Management	Works in partnership to agree a plan that patient has ownership of; uses reflective questioning to aid this if necessary	Establishes clear plan for management of long-term condition	Incompletely addresses long-term management	Does not arrange for admission of likely sickle cell crisis
Interpersonal skills	Maintains respectful and non-judgemental approach, working in partnership with patient; checks understanding	Explores patient's health beliefs and preferences	Does not adequately explore psychosocial aspect of presentation, including reasons for disengaging	Didactic style of consultation; talks down to patient

Trainer's comments

There are two main **priorities in this consultation**, which the examiners will be looking to you to address:

- Management of the acute presentation (i.e. a likely sickle cell crisis).
- Engagement with long-term management of her condition.

For management of the acute presentation, this patient has joint/bone pain in association with a temperature. In line with current NICE guidance (1), she should be admitted for an immediate assessment of a likely sickle cell crisis. All people with clinical features of a sickle cell crisis should be admitted to hospital unless they are:

- A well adult who only has mild or moderate pain and has a temperature of 38 °C or less.
- A well child who only has mild or moderate pain and does not have an increased temperature (2).

Your data gathering in this area should include some questions about the patient's current presentation and an examination of the chest, abdomen and musculoskeletal system.

She should be amenable to attending hospital if you can communicate clearly and sensitively the potential seriousness of her current condition.

In terms of **engagement with the long-term management of the condition**, the patient clearly has some element of denial here and there is much to suggest that she is disengaging with her long-term management. For example, she has missed two clinic appointments, she is not taking her medication reliably and she has missed the flu vaccine this year. Within your data gathering you should explore why she is disengaging like this and gauge her understanding of her condition. The journey from adolescence to adulthood can be a complex time for people with a chronic condition, and a complex interplay of personal and emotional factors can influence the individual's engagement with that chronic condition. There may be an element of **denial** here, which should be addressed.

It is also worth expanding on the **social situation**. Why is she attending without her mother this time? What are her feelings about her siblings not having the condition? Being a future medical student, has she read more about the condition than the usual patient of her age? Is she aware of the long-term prognosis/complications?

You need to engage with her as a doctor and arrange for her to see you again (whether she is admitted or not). Explain that you can re-refer her to the specialist outpatient clinic again if this is not arranged directly via the hospital team today.

A good candidate would be able to demonstrate strong **interpersonal skills** here, using this opportunity to engage with the patient in a way that is open and non-judgemental.

Looking at interpersonal skills, this is a case where some of Roger Neighbour's ideas would be pertinent (3):
- **Rapport building**: Establish this early with an open style of consulting.
- **Summarising**: Reflect back during your data gathering and your management plan.
- **Handing over**: Specifically with respect to your agreed plans for her long-term management.
- **Safety-netting**: This is less relevant as it is likely that an acute admission will be required.
- **Housekeeping**, even within CSA: If this or any consultation goes badly, take a deep breath and clear your head. You are allowed to have a bad consultation – good candidates will accept this and 'bounce back' for the next one.

One thing is for sure: the patient will not react well to being patronised by her doctor, but equally she needs to be challenged. Asking some reflective questions may be helpful here, such as 'Where would you like to see yourself next year?' or 'How would we need to manage your sickle cell disease to get there?'. It would be useful to discuss with your peers what sort of questions each of you would use here.

As well as addressing the patient's **follow-up** in clinic, it may be useful to arrange a review after her acute attendance to tie up any loose ends from this consultation, and to explore other areas that you may not have addressed fully today (such as contraception, vaccinations and so on).

References

1. National Institute for Health and Clinical Excellence (2012) *Sickle Cell Acute Painful Episode*. London: NICE. http://guidance.nice.org.uk/CG143
2. NICE Clinical Knowledge Summary. Sickle cell disease. http://cks.nice.org.uk/sickle-cell-disease
3. Neighbour, R. (2004) *The Inner Consultation*. 2nd rev. edn. Milton Keynes: Radcliffe Publishing.

Case C11

C11 Diabetes (telephone consultation)

Patient brief: Mr Pierre Riberry

You are a 47-year-old self-employed baker. You are a type II tablet-controlled diabetic who also suffers with high cholesterol and high blood pressure. You are compliant with your medications, which you know well (metformin three times a day, gliclazide twice a day, amlodipine, simvastatin and ramipril once a day).

You ate out a couple of nights ago at a local restaurant and the next morning you started to develop severe diarrhoea and vomiting. You are experiencing loose stools several times a day with abdominal cramps. These are thankfully easing when opening your bowels and they come in waves. They are not that severe. There is no mucus or blood in your stool. The vomiting is starting to ease (going only a few times a day) and you can keep water down but struggle to keep any food down; in fact, you haven't really eaten anything since then.

Because of this, you have stopped taking all of your diabetic medicines and have just taken the others. You do not routinely check your blood sugar, but do have a machine with you which you can check. You have never checked your urine for any sugar and do not have the facility to do so. You feel thirsty and weak but not faint and have no other symptoms (no loss of weight or blood in vomit or stool). You have not been travelling abroad recently.

You are currently staying at a friend's place near your work, but it's far from home and the surgery. You cannot afford to take any time off work as you are self-employed as a baker, and any time away from the shop floor is a loss of profit.

You are divorced with two children (aged 8 and 10) who live with your wife in France. You have to pay child allowance back to your ex, so money is tight. If the doctor suggests that you should not work, you explain that physically you can manage it and put up some resistance to the suggestion of time off. Being self-employed means you cannot claim any short-term sick benefit. If explained clearly enough and with some empathy towards your plight, you would be willing to let your friend run the bakery with clear instructions from you over the telephone. You would thus want to know when you could go back to baking.

Patient's opening remarks: '*I've got a really bad tummy, doc, and I need some advice please.*'

Patient's agenda: You are feeling a bit weak but want some advice from the doctor regarding how to get over this stomach bug. You are staying well out of the practice area and if offered an appointment to be seen in the practice, you kindly decline, as it's too far to travel without any toilet facilities along the way. You are not keen on any visit to A&E, if suggested, as you do not feel that ill and don't want any time off work (or not to be able to supervise your friend baking via a telephone).

EXAMINATION FINDINGS

If asked to check their blood glucose (BM), the actor says it is 14.2.

Reflection
Key points
- **Data gathering:** Rule out red flags (blood, travel, inability to hydrate, high fever, excruciating abdominal pain, mucus). Get the patient to perform a BM.
- **Management:** Encourage him to use fluids; regular checking of BM; stop metformin and ramipril but insist on him continuing with the other medications. Advise him not to go to work and also notify the health protection agency, given his profession. Safety-netting appropriately is especially important in telephone consultations.
- **Interpersonal skills:** It's important to establish the identity of the caller, but still to use open and closed questions appropriately. Encourage the patient to speak. Use empathy to convince him not to go back to work until 48 hours after the symptoms have resolved.

	Clear Pass	Pass	Fail	
Data gathering	Performs a BM over the telephone; asks if the patient can perform a urine ketone test	All red flags established, as well as occupation	No occupation established nor that the patient has stopped diabetic meds	
Management	Stops metformin and ramipril temporarily; books routine diabetic review when well	Checks BM; safety-netting; says cannot go to work until 48 hours after symptoms have resolved	Advice re fluids and re-starting medications; no advice re checking BM or safety-netting	
Interpersonal skills	Delivers information in bite-size chunks and summarises at the end	Picks up cues about work; safety-nets; shows empathy towards work	Fails to pick up cues, e.g. worries over finances/work	

Trainer's comments

This is a telephone consultation, so it is important to start by establishing that you have the **correct patient** on the phone; this can be easily done by confirming the patient's full name. The same advice applies about asking open questions first before honing in on a diagnosis of gastroenteritis by the use of closed questions.

It is important to establish that there are no **red flags** present (such as severe abdominal pain not eased by opening bowels; foreign travel; rectal bleeding; high fever; ability to maintain hydration; and mucus in stool). Once this is done, the doctor can be confident that this can

be safely managed on the phone; even if the doctor wanted to see the patient this would not be possible and, given the benign nature of the condition, insistence on seeing a local GP in another practice or attending A&E would be a waste of resources and probably inappropriate. Furthermore, sending stool cultures or trying to arrange bloods locally would be both difficult to do and a waste of resources.

The patient's **diabetes** does complicate things somewhat, but the main management will revolve around regular (at least once a day or if feeling unwell) blood sugar monitoring, adequate fluid advice and diabetic sick-day rules (i.e.

must carry on with usual diabetic medicines, with the exception of ramipril and metformin, which can potentially cause lactic acidosis in a dehydrated state). The latter is rare, so it's probably not essential for you to do well in the station. It would be useful to get him to check his BM while you're on the phone. Ideally, the patient would also be able to check for ketones in his urine, but given that he doesn't have this facility and his BM is not too high, this can be overlooked.

The patient being self-employed is another complicating factor. An infectious gastric illness is contagious and as a food handler he should not be at work for at least 48 hours after symptoms have resolved. His inability to obtain sick pay does make things harder, but empathising while pointing out that if one of his customers became sick he could get into trouble should help convince him of the merits of not going to work. You would need to inform the health protection agency out of courtesy, but this should not affect the patient, as it is merely for survelllance in his case. His

latest HBa1C is a little high, so asking him to book an appointment with the diabetic nurse when he is well would be worthwhile.

Safety-netting is especially important here – ask the patient to call back if there are any red flags: a very high blood sugar (e.g. 25) or if symptoms were not settling by a specific time (perhaps within a week or so).

Further Reading

Diabetes UK. Feeling ill: Information for young people with diabetes. http://www.diabetes.org.uk/Guide-to-diabetes/My-life/Kids/Me-and-my-diabetes/Getting-my-glucose-right/Feeling-ill

Patient UK leaflet on diabetes and inter-current illness. http://www.patient.co.uk/doctor/Diabetes-and-Intercurrent-Illness.htm

Public Health England. List of notifiable diseases. http://www.hpa.org.uk/Topics/InfectiousDiseases/InfectionsAZ/NotificationsOfInfectiousDiseases/ListOfNotifiableDiseases

Case C12

C12 Asthma (teenager)

Patient brief: Master Philip Hare

You are a 16-year-old student who has asthma. You have been asked to make an appointment to see the doctor as your medication review date is past. You think this will be a waste of time, as they generally don't do much and you are keen to get back to revise for your upcoming GCSEs.

You are not stressed, but have been putting yourself under a lot of pressure. This has led to you smoking a packet of cigarettes a day. This is something you admit to the doctor, but only if asked specifically. You are keen for your parents not to know and you will only open up more if the doctor reassures you that everything you say is confidential. Your parents are at work and you are an only child. Things at home and school are fine.

Your asthma has not been that well controlled of late. You need your blue inhaler a few times a day, especially if you are playing football. You have found that you cannot perform as well at football these days. If the doctor can convince you that you would breathe better by taking a new inhaler and giving up smoking, you could be convinced, but would not consider seeing someone about your smoking or giving up until after your exams in a month.

If asked, your breathing has not affected your sleep, but it has stopped you playing football and your chest has felt tight a few days of the week. You do not feel unwell currently and have not had a cough or fever. Your inhaler technique is good and you should be prepared to have a respiratory exam performed on you.

Patient's opening remarks: '*I was told to come and see you…*'

Patient's agenda: You think this will be a waste of time. You are worried that your parents may find out that you are smoking.

EXAMINATION FINDINGS

The candidate should be allowed to examine the patient. No clinical signs. Inhaler technique is good. PEFR is 330 l/min.

Reflection

Key points

- **Data gathering:** respiratory exam; smoking status; any stresses at home/school.
- **Management:** starting a steroid inhaler, giving smoking-cessation advice and advising on follow-up.

- **Interpersonal skills:** Use patient-friendly terms and a style appropriate to teenagers. Summarise and build rapport and empathy towards the patient's situation. Establish confidentiality clearly.

Suggested marking criteria

	Clear Pass	Pass	Fail	Clear Fail
Data gathering	Asks RCP three questions (or similar)	Respiratory exam, inhaler technique and smoking status; exam stress established	Basic respiratory exam, no inhaler technique or PEFR; social situation not enquired about	No smoking
Management	Spacer device prescribed	More detailed information on use of steroid inhaler and side effects; follow-up advised	Steroid inhaler started with minimal explanation; smoking-cessation advice	No changes to medication
Interpersonal skills	Delivers information in bite-size chunks and summarises at the end; empathy towards exam stress	Picks up cues about exam; discusses confidentiality; consults in a teenage-friendly way	Fails to pick up cues, e.g. worries over exam; does not cover confidentiality	Didactic style of consulting with no emotion shown towards the patient or his situation

---

Trainer's comments

Although the majority of this station is about asthma management, the impact of smoking and the **cause for it** (exam stress) should not be overlooked. The actor should not lead the patient down the path of a teenager who is stressed, but you should show some empathy towards what is a difficult time in their life. Explaining early on that everything that is discussed is confidential, while trying to encourage some help from an adult, may be prudent, but insisting on the latter is not appropriate. A 16-year-old can consent to treatment if they have capacity to do so, but cannot refuse treatment if it is in their best interests. Smoking-cessation treatment could loosely fit into the latter, but most sensible doctors would not break confidentiality just for smoking. Putting a 16-year-old off attending the practice would not be a good idea – they may never attend again.

Asking the **RCP three questions** (1) would help steer your **management** and establish that the patient is at moderate risk of an exacerbation, so something needs to be done today; that is, in the past month/week:

1 Has your asthma affected your sleep?
2 Have you had your usual asthma symptoms during the day?
3 Has your asthma affected your usual activities?

A routine chest examination, inhaler technique and peak expiratory flow rate (PEFR) measurement should be performed quickly to rule out a current exacerbation.

The **pharmacological management** will revolve around the introduction of a regular steroid inhaler. Explain that it works just within the lungs, and how it works (in a patient-friendly way: for example, 'it reduces swelling in the airways') and that its effects will take time to be seen. In terms of choice of device, another metered-dose inhaler (MDI) would be a sensible option (with a spacer for the steroid inhaler) given his good inhaler technique; this would prevent the need to learn about another device. It is good practice to advise the patient to rinse his mouth after using the steroid inhaler, which should be used twice a day regularly.

Regarding **smoking**, it would be sensible to advise that this is making his breathing worse and to use some rapport to suggest that his football would be better if he stopped smoking. Explaining that the best way to give up smoking is with help from an NHS service would complement this, but understanding that right now he is not keen to give up until after his exams would be important. Advising follow-up after his exams both for smoking and his asthma would be sensible.

Reference

1. Royal College of Physicians. Measuring clinical outcome in asthma. http://www.rcplondon.ac.uk/publications/measuring-clinical-outcome-asthma

Further Reading

Asthma UK. Inhaler device demonstrations for patients. http://www.asthma.org.uk/Sites/healthcare-professionals/pages/inhaler-demos

British Thoracic Society and Scottish Intercollegiate Guidelines Network (SIGN). British guideline on the nanagement of asthma. http://www.brit-thoracic.org.uk/Portals/0/Guidelines/AsthmaGuidelines/qrg101%20revised%202009.pdf

General Medical Council. 0–18 years: Guidance for all doctors. http://www.gmc-uk.org/guidance/ethical_guidance/children_guidance_index.asp

Case C13 📷

PATIENT

Name: Mr Joseph Riley
Age: 75
SH: Social drinker, never smoked
PMH: High cholesterol
DH: Simvastatin 40 mg nocte

C13 Acute red eye

Patient brief: Mr Joseph Riley

You are a 75-year-old retired carpenter who has high cholesterol that runs in the family. You take a tablet for it. You have come because you have a painful red right eye. It started a few hours ago. If asked, you had been feeling a bit unwell today with a cold-like illness and some nausea. As the day progressed, your right eye started to hurt and you noticed it had become red. It was never sticky and, if asked, your vision has become blurry as well as sensitive to light. You normally wear glasses only to read. You would like to know what the diagnosis could be and why it is so important to go to hospital today.

Patient's opening remarks: *'It's my eye, doctor, it's very painful and it looks very red.'*

Patient's agenda: You live alone and, if asked, you are worried about who will take care of your dog if you need to stay in hospital. If prompted by the doctor, there is a neighbour who could take care of him, but you would need to go back to your flat to give your dog to your neighbour. You got a lift to the doctor's from another neighbour. You do not have any money for a cab. You don't mind going to hospital, but you are keen for something to be done for your dog. You do not feel safe enough to walk back alone as you are afraid you may have an accident as you cannot see properly.

EXAMINATION FINDINGS

If asked, eye feels hard and looks red.
If asked, pupil does not react to light.

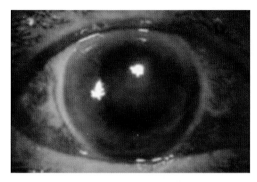

Figure 7.2 Source: From Wiley Ophthalmology at a Glance, p32

Reflection

Key points

- **Data gathering:** Recognising that this patient has acute angle closure glaucoma is key to insisting that he attend the hospital today. Likewise, establishing that the patient is not safe to leave alone is important.

- **Management:** Be flexible with transporting the patient to hospital and trying to understand his point of view, while ensuring that he gets to hospital as soon as possible.

- **Interpersonal skills:** Explore support at home and acknowledge that his dog's wellbeing is high on his agenda.

Suggested marking criteria

	Clear Pass	Pass	Fail	Clear Fail
Data gathering	Social circumstances, neighbour support	Safety of the dog being paramount to the patient	Painful red eye	Recently felt unwell
Management	Gives the patient options of how to get the dog looked after, but ensuring hospital admission ASAP	Comes up with idea(s) to organise care of the dog while ensuring hospital transfer	Ignores the patient's worries regarding the dog	Does not refer to hospital
Interpersonal skills	Takes a flexible approach, giving options	Empathetic and sensitive discussion over problems and ways to help	Fails to form rapport or be empathetic to circumstances	Fails to listen to patient's wishes

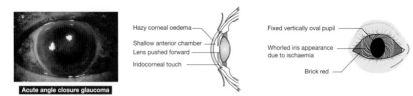

Acute angle closure glaucoma

Hazy corneal oedema
Shallow anterior chamber
Lens pushed forward
Iridocorneal touch

Fixed vertically oval pupil
Whorled iris appearance
due to ischaemia
Brick red

Figure 7.3

Trainer's comments

Recognising that this is an **ophthalmological emergency** as this patient has acute angle closure glaucoma is key to insisting that he attend the hospital today. Acute angle closure glaucoma is a sight-threatening condition that often presents with malaise and an acute painful red eye, mainly in the elderly. Examination may reveal a red eye that is hard, mid-dilated and unreactive to light. Urgent referral the same day to ophthalmology is required.

It is also important to establish that the patient is not safe to leave alone. Exploring support at home is central to this station, as well as acknowledging empathetically that his dog's wellbeing is very high on his agenda; in fact, it would prevent him from going direct to the hospital.

There are several valid management approaches in terms of helping him with arrangements to get to hospital today. Be flexible with transport – could he go via his home so that his dog can be given to the neighbour? Or perhaps you could contact the neighbour yourself so that they could pick up the keys from the patient now, or maybe you could even involve the RSCPA in the dog's care. The key here is being flexible and trying to understand the problem from the patient's point of view, while ensuring that he gets to hospital as soon as possible.

Further Reading

Patient UK. Information on acute angle closure glaucoma. http://www.patient.co.uk/doctor/angle-closure-glaucoma

Index

Page numbers in *italics* denote figures and **bold** to tables.

How to Pass the CSA Exam, First Edition. Imtiaz Ahmad, Raj Nair, Martin Block and Graham Easton.
© 2015 John Wiley & Sons, Ltd. Published 2015 by John Wiley & Sons, Ltd.